THE PROTEIN ADVANTAGE COOKBOOK

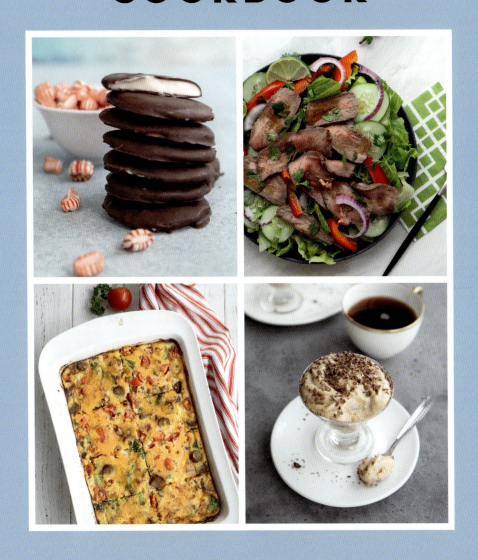

Quarto.com

© 2025 Quarto Publishing Group USA Inc.
Text and Photography © 2025 Carolyn Ketchum

First Published in 2025 by Fair Winds Press, an imprint of The Quarto Group,
100 Cummings Center, Suite 265-D, Beverly, MA 01915, USA.
T (978) 282-9590 F (978) 283-2742

Fair Winds Press titles are also available at discount for retail, wholesale, promotional, and bulk purchase. For details, contact the Special Sales Manager by email at specialsales@quarto.com or by mail at The Quarto Group, Attn: Special Sales Manager, 100 Cummings Center, Suite 265-D, Beverly, MA 01915, USA.

29 28 27 26 25   1 2 3 4 5

ISBN: 978-0-7603-9352-9

Digital edition published in 2025
eISBN: 978-0-7603-9353-6

Library of Congress Cataloging-in-Publication Data available.

Design and page layout: Laura Klynstra
Cover Image and photography: Carolyn Ketchum, @FoodDreamer

Printed in USA

The information in this book is for educational purposes only. It is not intended to replace the advice of a physician or medical practitioner. Please see your health-care provider before beginning any new health program.

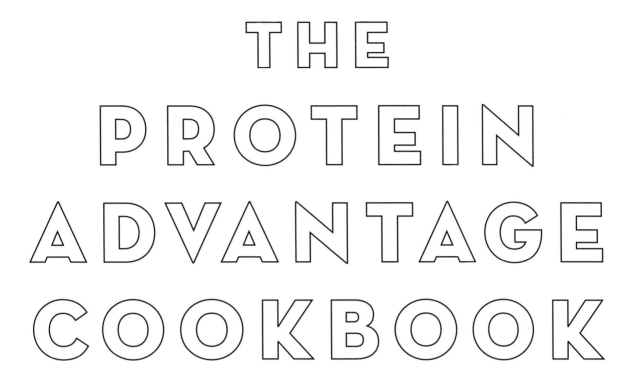

THE PROTEIN ADVANTAGE COOKBOOK

High-Protein, Low-Carb Recipes that Burn Fat,

Build Muscle, and Restore Metabolism

CAROLYN KETCHUM

Creator of @FoodDreamer

FAIR WINDS

CONTENTS

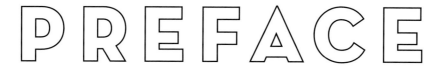

PREFACE

I am no stranger to major lifestyle changes and dietary overhauls. My own low-carb journey began over a decade ago, when I was staring down the barrel of type 2 diabetes. I had gestational diabetes with my third pregnancy and it seemed to resolve upon the birth of my daughter, but within a few months I found my blood sugar becoming increasingly difficult to control.

This came as quite a surprise to both my doctor and me, given my slender build, activity level, and lack of familial risk factors. Like many people with a serious health concern, I found myself with a choice: go on medication or try to address it through a lifestyle shift. As you might imagine, I chose the latter. And I have been successfully managing my blood sugar with diet and exercise for more than fifteen years.

But my journey is ongoing, and like any health journey, it is filled with twists and turns and a few bumps along the way. Different life stages inevitably bring their unique challenges and needs, and I have had to adapt and change course to meet those challenges.

The high-fat ketogenic diet served me well for many years, but as I approached menopause, I struggled with elevated glucose levels, particularly my fasting glucose. I also felt that the heavy-fat meals weren't sitting as well in my belly and made me feel somewhat sluggish. This was even noticeable to me at the gym, where I sometimes felt weak and lethargic.

Anecdotally, I was hearing from many readers, particularly women, that the high-fat approach caused weight loss stalls and other health concerns. So I began digging into the research on nutrition and aging. And as I tweaked my diet by increasing the protein and reducing the fat, I had greater success managing my blood sugar. I also found I gained more energy and even increased my lean muscle mass.

When I decided to write this book, I took a deep dive into the world of protein, nutrition, and healthy aging. I immersed myself in the latest research and literature, delving into medical journals and nutritional studies from across the globe. When I came up for air, I found myself utterly fascinated by the role protein plays in virtually every function of the human body—and thoroughly persuaded by the importance of consuming enough to support a healthy lifestyle.

I discovered far too much fascinating information and material to share in this cookbook, but I am ever more convinced that a high-protein approach is vital to good health on a low-carb diet—or any kind of diet, to be honest. Protein offers major health and physiological advantages at every stage of life, and it becomes increasingly important as we get older.

Are you ready to enjoy all that *The Protein Advantage Cookbook* has to offer? I am!

INTRODUCTION

What Is the Protein Advantage?

When people think of a low-carb, high-protein diet, they often picture bodybuilders and athletes consuming massive amounts of grilled chicken breast—and little else.

Let me assure you, this is not *that* kind of cookbook. Instead, I take a more practical and balanced approach, working from the assumption that better health is the ultimate goal of every reader. That goal might include weight loss, blood sugar management, building lean muscle mass, or simply having more energy for daily life. And all of us can take advantage of the health benefits of high-quality protein.

We all know dietary choices have a significant effect on health and vitality, but healthy food can be, and *should* be, more than just fuel for daily life. It should inspire us to sit down with family or friends and enjoy every bite that passes our lips. If our sustenance lacks flavor, if it fails to excite our taste buds and engage our mind, we are unlikely to stick with the program.

This is not a diet cookbook. It's also not a keto book or a "how to get shredded in 30 days" book. It is, however, a cookbook that offers tantalizing recipes for anyone who wants to increase protein, lower carbs, and feel more energetic.

The Protein Advantage Cookbook embraces the intersection of healthy choices and culinary innovation to motivate readers in the kitchen and beyond. As your guide, I offer a deep understanding of the transformative power of food. And the recipes contained herein are meticulously crafted to strike a balance between flavor and nutrition. Let's take advantage of delicious protein and healthier living.

Prioritizing Protein

The Protein Advantage Cookbook does not adhere to one single low-carb dietary philosophy, and everyone is welcome here. You can be keto and find value in this book. You can follow Atkins and find value in this book. You can be low carb or moderately low carb and find value in this book. You can count calories or watch your saturated fat intake and find value in this book.

The only requirement is that you prioritize protein. So what does that even mean? Let's dig in.

Your first consideration for any meal should be the protein content. What kind of protein will you have? How much protein do you want to consume? Is it high quality and easily absorbed?

Prioritizing protein also means being mindful of meeting your daily protein targets through a combination of meals and snacks. What that exact target is depends very much on the individual (see Determining Your Protein Goals, page 19).

Fat and carb consumption are secondary considerations, but that does not mean they are unimportant. You still need to be mindful of these nutrients and adjust them according to your dietary preferences and personal health goals.

In other words, you build the meal around the proteins. Your thought process when putting together meals and snacks should be something like this:

- What is my protein goal for this meal?
- What protein do I want to have?
- What low-carb sides or vegetables do I want to accompany the protein? How much should I have to stay within my carb limits?
- What fats do I need for cooking, flavor, and satiety?

When consuming the meal, you should also be mindful of eating all or most of the protein. If you feel like you are approaching fullness, focus on finishing the protein and leaving the added carbs and fats for another time.

The Evolution of Protein-Forward Low-Carb Diets

The low-carb diet world is neither static nor homogenous. Like any school of thought, it changes and evolves based on new developments and ideas. The very concept of "low carb" has no clear definition and encompasses a wide range of possible programs and dietary regimens. Anything between 20 and 130 grams of carbohydrates per day can be considered low carb; both are well below the current dietary guidelines of 225 to 325 grams, set by the US Departments of Agriculture (USDA) and Health and Human Services (HHS).

I have been creating low-carb recipes for well over fifteen years, long before "keto" exploded as a hot buzzword and the diet du jour. I have witnessed numerous transitions in that time frame. Indeed, my own approach to a healthy low-carb diet has undergone several transitions along the way.

At the height of its popularity, the ketogenic diet skewed heavily toward high fat consumption. Many keto and low-carb advocates promoted eating upward of 75 or 80 percent of daily calories from fat, keeping both carbs and protein quite limited. Some programs pushed for adding bacon, butter, and cheese to just about every meal. And quite a number of these experts promoted the idea that additional dietary protein would turn to glucose and halt weight loss and fat burning.

Although many devotees found success with these guidelines, others found that their weight loss stalled, or they even regained some weight. This was often the case as individuals got closer to their goal weights, when they had less body fat to lose.

I always found it hard to consume those extremely high levels of fat and tended to eat more protein than recommended. My goal wasn't weight loss but blood sugar control. And since I seemed to have little issue with a higher protein level, I always wondered about the veracity of these "strict keto" guidelines.

I can't say it came as any great surprise when I perceived a significant shift toward prioritizing protein. Over the past few years, more and more proponents have been focusing on a higher percentage of protein for both keto and low-carb diets. And many of those who cautioned that higher protein would stall weight loss have come to realize that this simply isn't true.

Prioritizing protein isn't some fad that's going to burn hot and fade fast. There is simply too much evidence to indicate that it is an integral piece of the health puzzle. And the protein-forward, low-carb approach has been shown to support health and vitality for people of all ages.

Should You Worry About Gluconeogenesis?

Gluconeogenesis literally translates to "the creation of new sugar" and refers to the body's ability to create glucose out of noncarbohydrate sources, such as lactate, lipids, and certain amino acids (proteins). It is a necessary biological process that occurs in all animals to maintain adequate blood sugar levels and avoid starvation. And it happens regardless of diet.

While gluconeogenesis does occur at a higher level in those consuming a low-carb or keto diet, this is simply because there are fewer carbs available to create glucose. Multiple studies and trials have shown that this does not translate into higher blood sugar, even in persons with type 2 diabetes. Certain tissues, such as the liver, require glucose to function, so gluconeogenesis is important for survival.

However, the idea that dietary protein can become glucose led a great many keto "experts" to caution against eating too much protein. The misconception that higher protein consumption would stall weight loss became widely accepted as fact. And it caused many people on keto diets to eat too little protein and to overconsume fats.

But as we see in this book, we need a higher level of protein to maintain lean muscle mass during weight loss, aging, and illness. Not eating enough protein, particularly during periods of fasting or ketosis, can cause muscle loss, weakness, and even impair the immune system.

How to Use This Book

The Protein Advantage Cookbook strives to inspire and educate. It is my fervent wish to provide readers with valuable information and new ideas as well as a wide array of tantalizing, protein-forward recipes. What you choose to do with the information contained herein is entirely up to you.

This book is not meant to offer a strict program or a diet regimen. There are many ways to approach a low-carb, high-protein diet, and there is no one-size-fits-all approach. I offer guidelines on how to determine your protein targets based on age, activity levels, and health goals (see page 20). I don't suggest specific carb limits, as such parameters depend heavily on personal needs and preferences.

A recent panel of experts put forth a standard definition of a low-carb diet as containing between 50 and 129 grams of dietary carbohydrates per day. Very-low-carb diets and ketogenic diets thus fall under 50 grams per day. This offers a broad spectrum of possibilities, and you will need to determine your own approach and carb tolerance.

Nutritional Information

Every recipe includes nutritional information—**calories**, **total carbs**, **dietary fiber**, **protein**, **fat**, and **saturated fat**—based on the specified ingredients. Optional ingredients are always included in the totals.

A recipe's carb count always refers to the **total** grams of carbohydrate—with one notable exception. The sweeteners I use most often (erythritol and allulose) have zero carb impact for the vast majority of people. Although technically they contain carbohydrates, they are metabolized by and eliminated from the body without ever raising blood glucose or insulin. For the purposes of a low-carb diet, they should not be counted as carbs, and I do not include them in the total carbohydrate grams.

> As someone with prediabetes/type 2 diabetes, my primary focus is managing my blood sugar levels, and I like to stay under 50 total grams of carbohydrates per day. This upper limit is based on what I observe on my glucometers as well as what makes me feel the most healthy and energetic.

If you wish to calculate net carbs, simply subtract the grams of dietary fiber from the grams of total carbohydrate.

I calculate nutritional information with a software program that relies on the USDA National Nutritional Database. This is the most comprehensive nutritional database in the country. I strive to be as accurate as possible, but errors do happen. I encourage you to calculate the nutrition independently. This is particularly important if you have a medical condition that requires strict adherence to macros.

Swaps and Substitutions

I recommend following the recipes as written, but I understand that food intolerances and ingredient availability sometimes necessitate substitutions. Wherever possible, I do my best to suggest appropriate swaps, but keep in mind that this may change the texture, flavor, and appearance of the finished dish. Also note that nutritional counts are calculated using the listed ingredients and will likely change with any substitutions.

Baking recipes require more precision than cooking recipes, and this is particularly true when using low-carb ingredients. Alternative sweeteners and flours behave very differently from each other, and substitutions can affect the results dramatically. Again, I suggest alternatives wherever possible, but I also recommend reading the articles I have written regarding how these ingredients behave. These can be found on my website at: alldayidreamaboutfood.com/faq/.

Quick Reference Icons

For those people with food allergies and intolerances, I've tagged the recipes in this book with easy labels. I have noted which recipes are free from dairy, nuts, and eggs as well as those recipes with options to make them free of common allergens. I've also noted which recipes are vegetarian.

Weights and Measures

Ingredients are listed in the Imperial style of volume measurements (cups and tablespoons), and since weighing ingredients can improve precision, particularly in baking recipes, metric equivalents are included for many ingredients.

CHAPTER 1

PROTEIN FOR HEALTHY LIVING

Let's step back in time for a moment to high school biology class. Amino acids, remember those? You likely learned that proteins are long chains of these smaller molecules. And amino acids are rightly considered the building blocks of life, as they are in every living thing, from microscopic organisms to great blue whales.

Protein is a major component of every single cell in our body—from muscles and bones to skin, hair, and nails. Proteins play a vital role in virtually every physiological function—from growth to digestion to fighting off disease. Even the synapses in our brains require protein to fire properly. That thought you just had? Yep, that's protein in action.

Why Protein Matters

To put it plainly, everything you are and everything you do requires protein. The very word *protein* comes from the Greek for "of primary importance" or "of first rank." We should consider it of primary importance in our daily diet too.

Protein Synthesis

The human body contains thousands of different kinds of protein, each with their own special function. Amazingly, however, all the protein in our body comprise only twenty amino acids. It is the sequence of the amino acid chain that determines the structure and function of the protein.

The body can produce some of these amino acids by itself through a process called *synthesis*. However, there are nine amino acids that mammals cannot synthesize directly: histidine, isoleucine, leucine, lysine, methionine, phenylalanine, threonine, tryptophan, and valine. Commonly referred to as "essential amino acids," these nutrients **must** be derived from dietary sources. And the best source of these nine essential amino acids is, of course, protein.

Our systems are constantly breaking down dietary protein into its amino acid components, sending those amino acids through the bloodstream and building them back into the proteins needed for a certain function.

This is a very rudimentary description of an astonishingly complex process; I hope it gives you a sense of just how important dietary protein is to our health and well-being. It's about so much more than pumping iron and building muscles. It's about quality of life.

Guidelines: What Is "Adequate" Dietary Protein?

Nutritional recommendations can be confusing and may even seem downright contradictory at times. It's important to remember that, like any research-based field, the science of nutrition is constantly evolving. New studies reveal new information, and new information spurs more studies.

Confusion arises when official guidelines don't reflect the most current research. Government agencies and professional associations are the source of official dietary guidelines. And we all know that government bureaucracy moves at the speed of a three-toed tree sloth.

Most dietary guidelines in the United States are issued by the National Academies of Sciences, Engineering, and Medicine. This includes the heavily relied upon Recommended Dietary Allowance (RDA), which is only revisited and revised every five to ten years. The current RDA for protein was set in 1941 and has remained unchanged since then.

With the RDA's target being a daily allowance, you are forgiven for assuming this means the amount of a nutrient you should realistically consume on a daily basis. As it happens, that assumption is incorrect. The RDA actually refers to the ***minimum amount*** you need for basic biological function.

In other words, the RDA is the minimum amount you need to avoid nutrient deficiency (a.k.a. malnutrition).

Digesting the Facts

- The Recommended Dietary Allowance (RDA) for protein does not reflect an optimal amount you should consume daily, but is instead the *minimum* you need for basic daily function.
- The current RDA for protein was established in 1941 and recommends 0.8 grams per kilogram of body weight for all adults, regardless of gender, age, activity level, or health status.
- Many experts have suggested that 1.2 to 1.6 grams provide a more appropriate target for protein consumption and improved health outcomes in most adults.

Surprised? Yes, I was too! The confusion is understandable because it is often misquoted and misrepresented as the **optimal amount** for daily intake. Many reputable sources make this same mistake, and some even suggest that anything above this amount is harmful to your health.

Currently, the RDA for protein stands at 0.8 grams per kilogram of body weight for adults over eighteen years of age. For an average adult weighing 160 pounds (72.6 kg), the RDA is 58 grams of protein. That is **the least amount** of protein that needs to be consumed to maintain their current level of lean muscle mass.

And this does not reflect other factors such as age, gender, metabolism, or activity level, all of which affect one's individual protein needs. Studies from the past twenty years indicate that most adults, particularly older individuals, could benefit from a significantly higher dietary protein intake. And yet the RDA for this vital nutrient has not changed in more than seventy years.

A growing body of research suggests that protein consumption in the range of 1.2 to 1.6 grams per kilogram of body weight results in improved health outcomes. And some sources recommend up to 2.4 grams for active adults. For our 160-pound (72.5 kg) average individual, that means anywhere from 87 to 174 grams of protein daily.

That's a big difference!

Benefits of Higher Protein

Many people embrace a low-carb diet as a means of promoting weight loss. Indeed, carbohydrate restriction as a tool for shedding body fat is well established. When compared to low-fat diets, study after study demonstrates that low carb is more expedient and sustainable.

A reduction in carbohydrates, almost by necessity, requires a corresponding increase in one or both of the other two macronutrients (fat and protein). And the evidence in favor of prioritizing protein is significant. This holds true for weight loss as well as myriad other health considerations.

- **Blood pressure:** Studies have shown a strong inverse relationship between protein consumption and developing high blood pressure. One study found that the highest protein intakes were associated with the greatest reduction in risk. And high-protein diets can help those who have hypertension.

- **Blood sugar:** It almost goes without saying that reducing carbs elicits better blood sugar control, but a corresponding increase in protein may be equally important. High-protein diets are associated with a lower risk of developing prediabetes, type 2 diabetes, and metabolic syndrome. There is also evidence that consuming more protein improves insulin resistance.

- **Body composition:** Higher-protein diets improve body composition by preserving lean muscle mass and reducing fat mass. This is particularly important during calorie-restricted diets. Studies that compare high-carb, low-fat diets to high-protein diets found that subjects lose about the same amount of weight, but those eating more protein lost more fat and less muscle. This is also true for intense athletic training. If energy expenditure exceeds dietary protein, greater muscle protein breakdown can result.

- **Injury:** Consuming higher amounts of protein can also improve and accelerate healing of wounds, fractures, and soft tissue injuries. The cells involved in the healing process require protein for proper function, as does the immune system to help ward off infection. And if the patient is bedridden or otherwise severely restricted, additional protein helps protect muscle mass.

- **Lean muscle mass:** Protein-rich diets help reduce or prevent muscle loss due to aging or illness (sarcopenia). And increased protein intakes are positively associated with improved muscle function in the elderly.

- **Lipid panels:** Contrary to some schools of thought, high-protein diets have also been shown to improve lipid profiles by decreasing triglycerides and increasing HDL (the good cholesterol). One analysis found that individuals who consume at least 1.1 to 1.5 grams of protein per kilogram of body weight had a reduced risk of developing cardiometabolic disease.

- **Weight loss:** High-protein diets promote satiety, making you feel fuller for longer. This is in part because a protein-rich meal regulates the hormones that control appetite, stimulating those that decrease hunger and suppressing those that increase it. This sense of fullness can last well beyond the meal itself and reduce consumption at subsequent meals, thereby reducing overall caloric intake.

Do note that *prioritizing protein* does not mean eliminating fat from our diet. Good-quality fats, both saturated and unsaturated, are vital to many biological functions, such as hormone regulation and vitamin absorption. Fats also help give our food flavor and make it more satiating—but because fat is more filling, it can impede our ability to consume enough dietary protein. A very-high-fat meal may make you feel too full to meet your protein goals, either for that meal or for the day. And eating both very high fat and high protein could lead to overconsumption and weight gain.

I found that as I increased my protein, my fat consumption decreased naturally. I don't count calories or fat grams; I simply prioritize protein and make it the center, the most important part, of every meal.

Did You Know?

The "second-meal effect" is a nutritional phenomenon whereby a previous meal has a significant impact on the digestive outcomes of subsequent meals. It is particularly noticeable in the postprandial glucose levels of both the first and second meals of the day. Many studies have shown that a high-protein breakfast can help keep blood glucose levels more stable throughout the day, even if subsequent meals are higher in carbohydrates. This appears to hold true for both healthy individuals and those with type 2 diabetes.

What About the Risks?

Many people have been scared away from increasing dietary protein because of purported health risks. The most pervasive is the notion that high-protein diets cause kidney damage. Many recent studies, though, have found this concern to be entirely unfounded in healthy individuals with no impaired renal function. Patients with pre-existing kidney disease are still advised to moderate their protein intake, in accordance with their doctor's advice.

Another prevalent concern is that high protein can adversely affect bone density. This too appears to be unfounded and based on incorrect data and conclusions. In fact, a recent review found a positive correlation between increased protein, calcium absorption, and bone mass. And higher protein may offer some protection against osteoporosis and reduce the risk of hip and other bone fractures later in life.

Similarly, a recent literature analysis found no direct correlation between increased dietary protein and cardiovascular disease or type 2 diabetes. Nor is there a correlation between high protein intake and colon or breast cancer. Once again, greater protein consumption may actually offer some protective effects on these health issues.

Protein Through the Ages

Forty may be the new thirty, but our body doesn't always agree. Our capacity to build and maintain muscle begins decreasing as early as our thirties, and the rate of decline accelerates with increasing age. By eighty, some adults will lose 40 to 50 percent of their muscle mass.

As we age, the ability to metabolize and synthesize protein into lean muscle mass decreases, a condition known as anabolic resistance. In other words, our body becomes less and less efficient at using the protein we consume to build or maintain muscle. And so it takes more dietary protein for an adult over fifty to build the same amount of muscle as an individual under thirty.

Many experts believe that doubling the RDA for protein provides a more appropriate target for optimal muscle health as we age. And this rate should be even higher for active adults or those who engage in strength training, as well as those recovering from serious illness or injury.

Yet studies from the past two decades indicate that a large percentage of adults are not consuming enough protein to maintain a healthy body into middle age and beyond. Given that many seniors are not even meeting the standard RDA of 0.8 gram per kilogram of body weight, we are clearly falling far short of protein needs. And in an aging population, that is cause for concern.

But the good news is that biology is not destiny; you don't need to resign yourself to a future of frailty in your later years. The actions you take now will help ward off problems in the future. Proper nutrition and exercise, particularly resistance strength training, can slow and even prevent age-related muscle loss.

And as the old adage goes, it's never too late to start. Take it from someone who embraced high protein and regular exercise later in life and has more muscle in her fifties than she ever did in her twenties and thirties!

Did You Know?

Not only does consuming more protein help you feel satiated, but doing so can actually boost your metabolism. Protein is significantly more *thermogenic* than either fat or carbohydrates, meaning it requires more energy to digest and assimilate the nutrients into the body. High-protein diets are associated with raised energy expenditures regardless of activity level.

Sarcopenia

Adults lose an estimated 3 to 8 percent of lean muscle mass every decade after the age of thirty. As with almost any health condition, muscle loss is severely affected by poor nutrition and a sedentary lifestyle. Unchecked, it often leads to *sarcopenia*, in which significant loss of muscle mass is accompanied by loss of strength and function.

This age-related condition causes much of the frailty and debilitation common in elderly adults, and it can contribute to other metabolic disorders such as insulin resistance, diabetes, and obesity. It even has a strong correlation to rheumatoid arthritis.

Exercise

While this book focuses primarily on the dietary aspects of healthy aging, I would be remiss not to mention the importance of exercise. The relationship between protein consumption and physical activity is a highly synergistic one. To engage in one without the other is addressing only part of the equation. Like any biological process, the interplay between the two is complex and multifaceted, but it's worth trying to understand on a basic level.

The human body constantly breaks down muscle tissue (muscle protein breakdown, or *catabolism*) and builds it back up again with new amino acids (muscle protein synthesis, or *anabolism*). You maintain lean muscle mass when these two processes are equal (*net protein balance*). You build muscle when the rate of synthesis exceeds the rate of breakdown (*net protein positive*), and you lose muscle mass when the rate of breakdown exceeds that of synthesis (*net protein negative*).

- Protein consumption helps stimulate muscle protein synthesis (net positive).
- Exercise stimulates muscle protein synthesis but also causes muscle protein breakdown. The rate of synthesis is typically higher than the rate of breakdown (net positive).
- A protein-rich meal consumed after exercise can help suppress muscle protein breakdown (net positive).
- Inactivity reduces muscle protein synthesis and can contribute to muscle protein breakdown (net negative).
- Inadequate dietary protein contributes to muscle protein breakdown (net negative).

Together, diet and exercise create a positive feedback loop, which helps build lean muscle mass exponentially faster than either can alone. On the flip side, lack of exercise and a protein-poor diet creates a negative feedback loop in which lean mass is degraded ever more quickly.

Resistance exercise is widely considered the most efficacious for building and/or maintaining lean muscle mass. This does not have to mean hitting the gym and lifting heavy weights. Simple body weight exercises, such as push-ups, sit-ups, squats, and lunges, can be extremely effective. And resistance bands provide an easy and inexpensive way to work out at home.

Anabolism: The creation of larger structures out of smaller units. In this case, the building of muscle (muscle protein synthesis) from smaller amino acids.

Catabolism: The breakdown of larger structures into their smaller components. Digestion of food is considered catabolism as is muscle protein breakdown.

Determining Your Protein Goals

There is no magic formula that calculates exactly how much daily protein we should consume. Everyone differs in body composition, activity level, age, and health status, all of which are important considerations. And personal health goals such as weight loss or muscle building add complexity.

Did You Know?

Anabolic resistance is the term used to describe the decreasing ability to synthesize protein from our daily diet as we age. Studies comparing healthy men of all ages have found that older individuals must meet a higher threshold of protein **in a single meal** to turn on an anabolic, or muscle-building, response. While a man of twenty-two can consume 15 to 20 grams of protein and efficiently use it toward muscle building and maintenance, a man of seventy will need to eat 25 to 35 grams to elicit the same physiological response. Most experts advise anyone over fifty to eat at least 25 grams of protein per main meal to turn on an anabolic response to feeding.

Menopause and Muscle Loss

Lean muscle loss for women accelerates as they approach and enter menopause. In female bodies, estrogen is one of the hormones that helps stimulate muscle growth and function. As estrogen declines, so too does the anabolic response from diet and exercise. Thus, postmenopausal women face an even greater challenge in maintaining healthy bodies as they age. And protein consumption is key to overcoming this challenge. One study found that women who ate a higher-protein diet—defined simply as higher than the RDA—had greater upper body strength, lower body mass, and better body composition than those who did not. Other studies have found high-protein diets (1.2 grams per kilogram of body weight) facilitated weight loss and were positively correlated with lean body mass.

Rather than focusing on an exact amount, try aiming for a range to fall within. This gives you some leeway to experiment on increasing your intake and timing to find what works best for you. Consider keeping a journal or log of meals and make a note of how you feel after high-protein meals.

We have already established that the RDA for protein is far too low for most adults, regardless of age, gender, and activity level. Research suggests that a better starting place is 1.2 to 1.6 grams per kilogram of body weight. From there, consider adjusting based on the following variables. Keep in mind there is a great deal of intersectionality here. You may fall into two or more of these categories, so start with a wider range and narrow it as you find what suits your needs.

- **Over 30:** Aim for at least 1.2 grams.
- **Over 50:** Aim for the higher end of 1.6 grams.
- **Moderate activity level:** Aim for 1.4 to 2 grams.
- **Intense activity level/heavy lifting:** Aim for 1.6 to 2.4 grams.
- **Muscle maintenance:** Aim for the range based on your level of activity.
- **Muscle building:** Use the heavy lifting range and aim for the high end.
- **Weight loss:** Aim for 1.6 to 2.0 grams per kilograms of your goal body weight while maintaining at least a caloric deficit. Using your goal weight is important because your current weight may overestimate protein, particularly if you have a lot of weight to lose.

- **Pregnancy and breastfeeding:** Aim for 1.2 to 1.9 grams; please always consult your doctor on any dietary changes and approaches during pregnancy and postpartum.
- **Postmenopausal:** Aim for at least 1.6 grams and increase the amount if trying to lose weight or build muscle.

Case Study

Using myself as an example, let's walk through how this might work:

- I am in my fifties and postmenopausal, so I feel I need to start with a base of at least 1.6 grams per kilogram of body weight.
- I am very active, do plenty of strength training, and don't want to lose weight. I would like to maintain the muscle I have and possibly build more. So, my range should be higher than 1.6 grams and toward the 1.8 to 2.4 grams range.
- Additional considerations: I have prediabetes and manage it entirely through diet and exercise. I keep my carbs quite low to keep blood sugar under control. Thus, protein is a vital source of nutrition and energy for me.
- I weigh about 115 pounds (52.2 kg) and I am 5'4" (163 cm) tall.

$$115 \div 2.2 = 52.3 \text{ kg}$$

$$52.3 \times 1.8 = 94 \text{ grams (low end)}$$

$$52.3 \times 2.4 \text{ grams} = 126 \text{ grams (high end)}$$

Based on this, I aim to consume 100 to 130 grams of protein per day. Some days I hit the low end; some days I hit the high end. Some days life happens and I don't hit my target. That's to be expected. I don't let it worry me because I know I can get back on track quickly and easily.

CHAPTER 2

MAXIMIZING YOUR PROTEIN INTAKE

A protein is a protein is a protein, right? Well, not exactly. The number you see on the nutritional panel on the back of the package doesn't tell the full story. When it comes to increasing your protein intake, there are several important considerations.

Digestibility: How much of the protein is actually digested by the human gut

Absorption rate: How quickly the digested protein is absorbed into the bloodstream

Bioavailability: How much of the protein is absorbed after digestion and reaches the target tissues to be utilized

☐ Find some delicious recipes for inspiration (you bought this book, so check!)

☐ Start at breakfast

☐ Aim for 25 to 35 grams per main meal

☐ Consider the source

☐ Spread it out

☐ Fuel up after workouts

☐ Supplement/snack as needed

In other words, it's complicated. And it becomes even more complicated when other nutrients, like fat and carbohydrates, are consumed concurrently, as they can slow digestion and absorption.

Best Sources of Protein

On the whole, animal proteins give you the most bang for your buck. Meat, poultry, fish, eggs, and dairy all have much higher digestibility and absorption rates and greater overall bioavailability than plant-based proteins. They also contain more protein per serving than their plant-based counterparts, so you don't need to eat nearly as much to meet your targets. As a result, animal proteins are typically considered of higher quality for sustaining our biological functions.

In fact, whey protein, which is found in cottage cheese, yogurt, and, of course, whey protein powder, is one of the most easily digested and absorbed forms of protein. It also contains high levels of leucine, a branched chain amino acid that promotes the most anabolic response. This makes it a great choice for anyone trying to maintain or build muscle mass.

None of this is meant to suggest you should focus all your efforts on a single protein source, nor that you should dismiss plant sources as unimportant or of low quality. As with any healthy diet, consuming a wide variety of foods not only keeps things more interesting but also gives you the benefit of many other important vitamins and minerals.

All proteins have varying amounts of essential amino acids, and our bodies use these amino acids for different functions at different times. It's not just our muscles, but every system in our body that utilizes these vital nutrients. Eating a variety of protein-rich foods helps us maximize the full amino acid profile.

Protein/Carbs per 100 grams (3½ ounces)

	Calories	Fat	Protein	Carbs
Broccoli, raw	39	0 g	3 g	6 g
Chicken breast, boneless, skinless, raw	106	2 g	23 g	0 g
Cottage cheese, low-fat	82	2 g	11 g	4 g
Eggs, large, whole	143	10 g	12 g	1 g
Garbanzo beans (chickpeas), canned, drained and rinsed	137	3 g	7 g	20 g
Greek yogurt, plain, low-fat	73	2 g	10 g	4 g
Hemp seeds, hulled	553	49 g	32 g*	9 g
Lean ground beef, 90/10, raw	176	10 g	20 g	0 g
Quinoa, cooked	120	2 g	4 g	21 g
Salmon (Pacific), raw	131	5 g	22 g	0 g
Tofu, raw, firm	144	9 g	17 g	3 g

Source: USDA Database

*While hemp seeds may seem like a great source of protein, you really don't want to eat 100 grams (3½ ounces) in one sitting—that would be a lot of calories and fat!

Vegans and Protein Consumption

People who follow a plant-based diet must consider the digestibility of the proteins they choose. For most whole plant foods, such as legumes or quinoa, digestibility ranges from 75 to 80 percent compared to whole animal sources. However, proteins that are isolated and extracted from plant sources, such as soy protein isolate, are much better digested and absorbed. This is compounded by the fact that plant-based proteins don't elicit as strong an anabolic response as animal sources. To compensate for these issues, many experts recommend eating at least 10 percent more plant-based protein to meet health goals.

Complete vs. Incomplete Proteins

You may have heard various protein sources referred to as "complete" or "incomplete." Complete proteins contain adequate amounts of all nine essential amino acids, whereas incomplete proteins may be very low or even lacking in some of the essential nine.

With the exception of gelatin and collagen, all animal protein sources have the complete amino acid profile. Alternatively, most plant-based sources are incomplete. Soy, quinoa, hemp seeds, and chia seeds are exceptions to this rule.

Does that mean you should eat only complete proteins and ignore the rest? Human nutrition is never quite so black and white. After all, it's not like our body ignores the nutrients in a food source simply because it's not classified as "complete." There is still plenty of good nutrition to be had, and our body still breaks down the amino acids present and puts them to good use.

You can also combine incomplete proteins with complementary foods that contain the missing amino acids. For example, collagen is incomplete because it doesn't contain any tryptophan (yes, the very same thing that makes you sleepy after a big turkey dinner). But you know what does contain plenty of tryptophan besides turkey? Chocolate. And peanut butter. And eggs! That means a recipe like the Deep-Dish Brownies (page 197) can be considered a complete source of protein.

You don't even need to combine the amino acid sources in the same meal as long as you eat them throughout the same day. So consider this another plug for eating a wide variety of protein foods, along with other healthy, low-carb foods, to get a balanced amino acid profile.

Timing and Distribution

The standard American diet skews toward carb-heavy meals in the morning, with greater protein consumption in the evenings. A low-carb, high-protein diet requires a significant shift in this pattern. And many sites and experts advise that you try to distribute your protein intake evenly throughout the day, eating 25 to 35 grams of protein at breakfast, lunch, and dinner.

The justification for this is the oft-quoted advice that we can only absorb 25 to 35 grams of protein from a single meal. But this may not be quite the open-and-shut case it appears to be. Although some studies indicate that an even distribution maximizes protein synthesis, others find that distribution patterns matter far less than total daily intake. Additionally, one recent study suggests that, for those engaging in strength training, there is no upper limit in the ability to absorb protein from one meal.

In other words, it's complicated. Sensing a theme yet?

There is something to be said for the even distribution approach, especially when trying to increase overall protein intake. For many people, it's not easy to eat large amounts of protein in one sitting. And starting earlier in the day helps ensure you meet the daily protein goals. As someone with a relatively small appetite in one sitting, this approach works best for me; however, if eating one or two larger meals per day works better for you, there is no need to adopt a whole new eating pattern. Focus instead on the total daily intake, making sure to consume at least one meal with sufficient protein to meet the target goal.

Exercise and Protein Timing

If you exercise regularly, you've likely heard that you should eat protein soon after working out. This advice is based on the idea that our body is primed to build muscle in the first 30 to 60 minutes after exercise. Many experts refer to this as the "anabolic window."

But recent studies have challenged this notion and indicate that the post-exercise recovery window should not be so narrowly defined. The anabolic effects of resistance training last far longer than 60 minutes and depend heavily on the individual, the kind of training, and what they have eaten in the previous 24 hours. The evidence suggests that most individuals benefit from eating a protein-rich meal within 3 to 4 hours of working out.

There also appears to be little difference between pre- and post-workout protein consumption. While the traditional advice leans heavily toward post-exercise, eating before exercise is just as beneficial for muscle building. And, once again, the most important number to concern yourself with is the total daily protein intake.

Digesting the Facts

Incomplete protein sources should not be dismissed as irrelevant or ineffective. When combined with other foods, they can provide a full amino acid profile.

Protein Supplementation

Protein supplementation is a multibillion dollar industry. Shakes, bars, cookies, chips, cereal, powders . . . you name it, somebody has added protein to it. And every brand has its celebrity or athlete endorsements, telling you why it's the best protein supplement on the market. So it begs the question: Do you really need all these high-protein products to be healthy?

The short answer is no. You can get all the protein you need from your daily diet, even when significantly increasing your intake. That said, sometimes a little protein supplementation is convenient, tasty, and can fill in any nutritional gaps.

I started experimenting with protein powder early in my journey because I found it improved the texture of my low-carb baked goods. I found it easy to tweak those recipes when I decided to prioritize protein. Being able to grab a protein muffin or an energy bite helps me stay on track when life gets hectic.

As with any food, quality matters. There are many kinds of protein supplements and thousands of different brands, so read the labels. Make sure they don't contain added sugars or other unhealthy additives. And use them primarily as snacks or easy ways to add a little more protein. In other words, use them in *addition to*, rather than as *a replacement for*, well-rounded high-protein meals.

Protein Powders in Cooking and Baking

In this book, I focus on protein powders and how to use them in recipes. Once again, there is a dizzying array of choices.

Animal-Based Protein Powders

- Beef protein isolate
- Bone broth protein
- Casein protein
- Collagen protein
- Egg white protein
- Whey protein

Plant-Based Protein Powders*

- Hemp protein
- Peanut protein
- Pea protein
- Pumpkin seed protein
- Rice protein
- Soy protein

*Plant-based powders are often blends to provide a complete protein profile. Keep in mind that many plant-based proteins have a grayish or greenish hue, which can affect the appearance of a recipe's results.

When choosing a protein powder, be sure to look at the ingredient list and nutritional label carefully. Some contain added sugars, artificial sweeteners like aspartame, or fillers like maltodextrin. Try to stick to brands that have fewer than 3 grams of carbs per serving and use natural flavors and sweeteners like stevia or monk fruit. Be sure to make note of any allergens that may cause issues.

Please also note that different protein powders behave very differently in baking, and substitutions can affect your results. Whey protein, egg white protein, and plant-based protein can usually be used interchangeably, but not always. Collagen protein, bone broth protein, and beef isolate protein powders are similar to each other, but behave very differently from whey or egg white powders (more on this in chapter 3).

Additionally, more is not always better when it comes to adding protein to your low-carb baking. Too much whey or egg white powder makes baked goods very dry. Too much collagen can cause the recipe to become gummy and dense. And the flavors of these protein powders can sometimes be overpowering.

The recipes contained in this book have been thoroughly tested using the ingredients and amounts listed. It is beyond the scope of this book to test every possible variation. Where possible, however, I have given suggestions for other options and my educated guess on how they will work.

If you plan to purchase only one kind of protein powder, I recommend unflavored whey or egg white powder. These have the broadest applications across recipes. You can always add flavor and sweetener to a recipe, but you can't remove it once it's there.

Did You Know?

Whey protein is one of the best sources of the branched chain amino acid leucine. Of all the amino acids, leucine elicits the greatest anabolic response, thereby increasing muscle protein synthesis.

Whey protein powder sometimes gets a bad rap in the low-carb world because it can cause a spike in insulin. Some people assume this leads to hyperinsulinemia (higher than normal levels of insulin in the bloodstream) and eventually to insulin resistance. However, studies show that whey protein actually helps regulate and decrease blood sugar levels, both in healthy people and those with type 2 diabetes.

Besides reducing postprandial glucose levels, increased insulin helps suppress muscle protein breakdown. Additionally, insulin helps transport amino acids into muscle tissue, increasing muscle protein synthesis.

CHAPTER 3

STOCKING YOUR LOW-CARB, HIGH-PROTEIN PANTRY

Preparation is the key to success on any healthy diet. We live in a high-carb world, where sugar and gluten are all around us all the time. It can be hard to resist when it's staring you down at every event, every get-together, and even the office breakroom. You are far more likely to succumb to temptation when you don't have a tasty array of low-carb, high-protein options on hand.

So take some time to evaluate your pantry, fridge, and freezer. Stock up on ingredients that help you create easy meals and snacks. Consider doing some meal planning and meal prep. Search out and save some tempting recipes to try. Make big batches of your favorites and freeze them for times when life gets overwhelming.

Have fun, embrace it, and know that you may have some false starts, some slipups, and some days where you get off track. We all do. The trick is to shake it off, avoid beating yourself up, and get right back on the horse.

Proteins

As we already discussed, meat products are some of the highest quality and bioavailable sources of protein. But, like any food, quality can suffer from overprocessing and additives. It's best to limit processed and cured meats and check sausages and premade burgers or meatballs for unnecessary ingredients.

Fish, Meat, Poultry	Dairy and Dairy Alternatives	Plant-Based Proteins
Fish	Cheeses: Cheddar, cottage, cream cheese, dairy-free cream cheese, mozzarella, parmesan; other cheeses	Almonds
Shellfish	Dairy-free yogurt	Chia seeds
Beef	Greek yogurt*	Flaxseed
Bison	Sour cream	Hemp seeds
Lamb	Unsweetened nut and seed milks	Peanuts
Pork		Pumpkin seeds
Chicken		Sesame seeds
Eggs		Soy products (edamame, tofu)
Turkey		Sunflower seeds

*In recipes using Greek yogurt, you will see references to "high-protein yogurt." Plain Greek yogurt is much higher in protein than traditional yogurt, but some brands are specifically high protein and low carb, such as Too Good and Chobani Zero Sugar. Try to choose yogurt with the highest amount of protein and the fewest carbs, without any added sugars.

For the dairy-free crowd, Kite Hill has a high-protein almond milk yogurt that is relatively low in carbs too!

As for how lean the meat is, the choice is yours. Keep in mind that meats with a high fat content will have a slightly lower protein content and will fill you up more. Fat adds flavor and increases satiety, but too much can prevent you from meeting your protein targets.

Produce

Not all vegetables are low in carbohydrates, so make sure you have a good array of lower-carb options to choose from. Listed here are the vegetables most used in this book.

And regarding fruit, although you need to be mindful of serving sizes, fruit can be part of a healthy low-carb diet. I've even been known to work a bit of apple or peach into my recipes. Listed following are the fruits I use most in this book.

Low-Carb Vegetables	Low-Carb Fruits
Asparagus	Avocados
Bell peppers	Blackberries
Broccoli	Blueberries
Brussels sprouts	Cranberries
Cabbage	Lemons
Cauliflower	Limes
Chile peppers	Raspberries
Cucumbers	Strawberries
Green beans	Tomatoes
Lettuce	
Mushrooms	
Radishes	
Sugar snap peas	
Zucchini	

Fats and Oils

When stocking your pantry, you don't need all of the oils listed here, but having a few options goes a long way for keto cooking and baking.

- Butter
- Ghee
- Mayonnaise
- Oils: Avocado, coconut, olive, sesame (toasted and untoasted)

Baking Supplies

I am well known for my advanced skill in low-carb baking and for pioneering methods to mimic the taste and texture of sugary, high-carb treats. Baking with low-carb, high-protein ingredients, however, is far from intuitive, as they behave very differently from flour and sugar.

Understanding these differences is vital to the results, so it warrants a brief discussion. I have written extensively about these subjects in other places, so be sure to check out the information on my website for a more in-depth discussion.

Low-Carb Flours

Almond flour and coconut flour are, perhaps, the most recognized and widely available low-carb alternatives to wheat flour. You can now find them in almost every grocery store, often in the baking aisle. And they are the ones I rely on most in this cookbook.

Although they are both very useful for low-carb recipes, they behave in vastly different ways. Coconut flour and almond flour are as different from each other as they are from wheat-based flours. So be aware that you cannot substitute one for the other with any measure of success.

Other nut and seed flours/meals are more similar to almond flour in overall texture and behavior. However, they are rarely as finely ground, which can affect the consistency and appearance of the finished recipe. Pumpkin seed meal is a great nut-free alternative to almond flour and has 11 grams of protein and only 4 grams of carbs per serving—but it does have a slightly greenish color.

All of these ingredients differ from wheat flour in that they lack gluten. Besides being a common allergen, gluten is responsible for the structure of conventional baked goods, helping them rise and hold their shape. We can overcome the absence of gluten through other means, but this is, in part, why low-carb baking is so different from traditional baking.

Please note that the recipes in this cookbook utilize blanched almond flour, so the brown skins have been removed from the almonds. Natural almond flour contains the skins, is coarser in texture, and produces a heavier baked good.

Making Your Own Nut and Seed Flours

Although you can rarely get homemade nut and seed flours as finely ground as the commercial varieties, it does make them more accessible and less expensive to grind them yourself. I make my own sunflower seed and pumpkin seed flours frequently.

You can use a food processor or blender, but I like to use a small coffee grinder. I recommend sifting the ground flour through a sieve to separate the more finely ground pieces from larger ones, then returning the bigger pieces to the grinder to get them more finely ground.

One cup (weight varies) of seeds or nuts usually makes about 1¼ cups (weight varies) of flour when freshly ground, but the flour decreases in volume a little over time as it compacts. I recommend making more than you need and measuring it after grinding.

Low-Carb Sweeteners

It is beyond the scope of this book to go into detail about the vast array of low-carb sweeteners on the market these days. A new one seems to appear at least every few months. Finding suitable alternatives to sugar is big business in our sweet-loving society.

All these sweeteners will promise you that they taste and bake "just like sugar!" But having tested a great many of them, I can assure you that not a single one does. They each have their advantages and disadvantages, and this is something I have written about extensively on my website.

For the recipes in this book, I use primarily erythritol and allulose-based sweeteners, in both granular and powdered (confectioners'-style) forms. Both are useful sweeteners, but it is important to understand that they behave very differently from one another. Erythritol can provide a crisp texture, whereas allulose will make things softer. In some cases, a substitution will make very little difference to the outcome, whereas in other recipes, swapping sweeteners will end in disaster.

In the recipes that follow, I have tried to be as specific or as general as the situation demands. In cases where multiple sweeteners work, I simply mention "sweetener." In recipes that rely on a particular kind of sweetener for flavor or consistency, I specify what it is and why it's important. I do not use sucralose or other artificial sweeteners that are not found in nature, so I cannot guarantee results if you choose to use them.

Protein Powders

I have long used protein powder in my low-carb baking, as it helps gluten-free baked goods rise properly and have a lighter, fluffier texture. I always recommend having at least one kind on hand, but they are even more important when you are trying to create high-protein desserts and snacks.

I dig into the various kinds of protein powders and how to use them in recipes a bit more in chapter 2. If you plan to purchase only one kind of protein powder, I recommend unflavored whey or egg white powder. These have the broadest application across recipes.

Specialty Ingredients

Although I try hard to stick to basic and readily available ingredients in my recipes, I also want to provide you with the best cooking and baking experience. That sometimes means using specialty ingredients to help get the right taste and texture. These are the ones I use most in this book:

Cocoa butter: I often use a little cocoa butter to aid in melting chocolate for dipping desserts like Coconut Candy Bars (page 210). Because cocoa butter is solid at room temperature, the chocolate coating is less melty, but you can also use a little coconut oil.

Don't Be Fooled!

Many sugar alternatives bill themselves as "monk fruit sweetener," which can be very confusing for new low-carb bakers. Pure monk fruit (*lo han guo*) is a highly concentrated extract made from a fruit found in China—a mere ½ teaspoon of this extract can sweeten an entire recipe that serves twelve people. Most "monk fruit sweeteners," though, are really erythritol (or sometimes allulose) in disguise. If you read the label on the package, you will see that the first ingredient is one of the bulk sweeteners. Since both erythritol and allulose are only 70 percent as sweet as sugar on their own, brands add a small amount of monk fruit extract to make it sweeter. It's a bit of a marketing gimmick, to be honest!

Cocoa powder: Cocoa powder isn't really a specialty ingredient since it's readily available, but it's worth discussing which cocoa powder you want to look for. I almost always recommend Dutch-process cocoa, which is treated with an alkaline solution (potassium bicarbonate) to help neutralize the natural acidity. This kind of cocoa powder has a deeper color, more chocolate flavor, and it mixes in better with other ingredients. Natural cocoa powder is lighter in color and doesn't dissolve as well in liquids or batters. And while the term "natural" may make you think it's healthier, it just refers to the fact that there is no alkali added during processing.

Extracts and flavorings: I love having a selection of flavors to add to snacks and baked goods. Besides vanilla extract, I like to keep almond, caramel, coconut, hazelnut, and lemon on hand. And since bananas aren't very low carb, I keep banana extract on hand for recipes like the Banana Bread Mug Cakes (page 71).

Glucomannan or xanthan gum: Both of these powders are useful as thickening agents for broths, gravies, and sauces. I find that glucomannan, a fiber derived from konjac root, blends more easily and doesn't clump as much as xanthan gum.

Grass-fed gelatin: You can usually purchase envelopes of gelatin at the grocery store, but I prefer to use healthier, grass-fed gelatin powder. It mixes into liquids more easily and is great for recipes like the Vanilla Blueberry Panna Cotta (page 205). Brands like Vital Proteins or Great Lakes Wellness are good options.

Low-carb chocolate: There are any number of great brands that make sugar-free chocolate bars or chocolate chips. You can often find them on grocery store shelves in the baking aisle or the natural foods aisle.

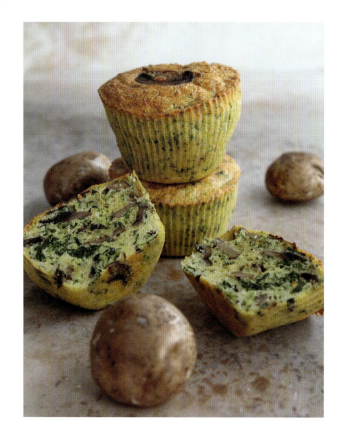

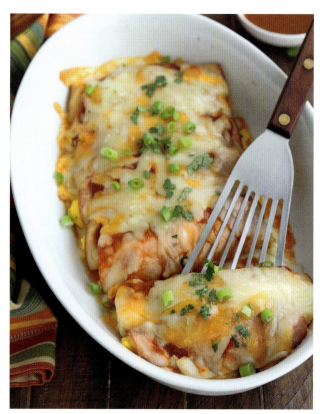

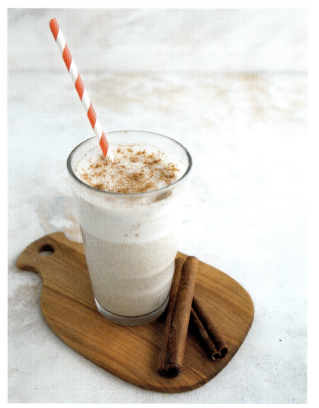

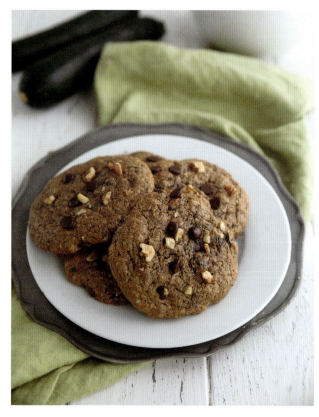

CHAPTER 4

BREAKFAST

Kick your day into high gear with these protein-packed breakfast recipes. Getting at least twenty-five grams of protein early on helps provide the energy to tackle whatever the day throws at you. And when you start off on the right foot, you're more likely to want to see things through on a positive note.

Try the Garlic and Herb Scrambled Eggs (page 38) or the Breakfast Enchiladas (page 43) for a savory start to your day. Or make a big batch of Cottage Cheese Waffles (page 56) and pair them with a few of the Turkey Breakfast Sausage patties (page 48). Many of these recipes are ideal for prepping ahead, so you won't be left scrambling on a busy weekday. But you can always whip up the Hot Maple Cereal (page 62) or the Banana Bread Mug Cakes (page 71) in a pinch!

If you prefer to work out first thing in the morning, consider a smaller protein snack with a larger meal afterward. However you like to break your fast, these high-protein options will keep you fuller for longer.

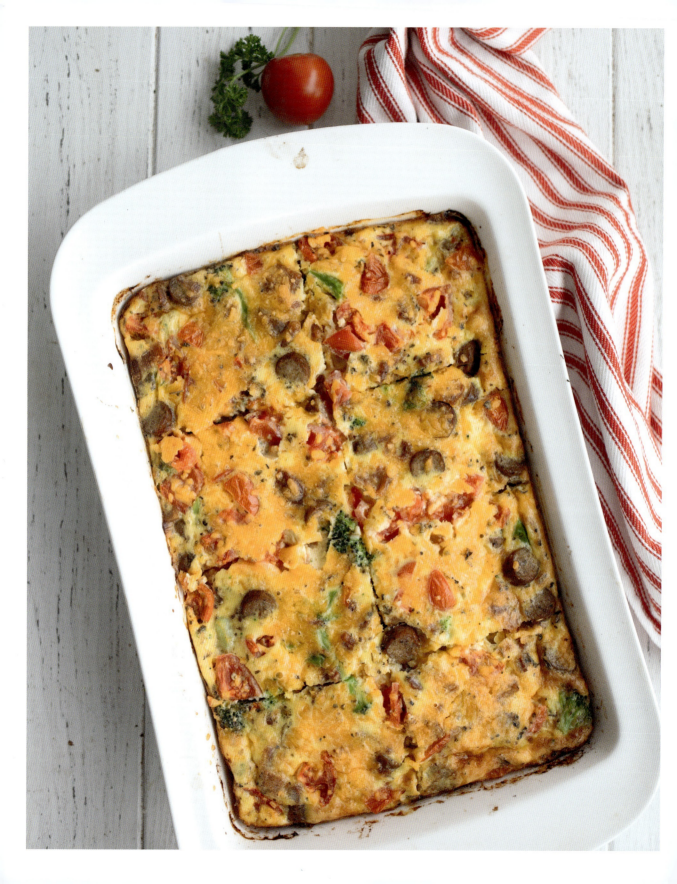

Loaded Breakfast Casserole

This hearty breakfast casserole is locked and fully loaded with protein! Packed with eggs, meat, and low-carb veggies, it makes an ideal high-protein brunch. It's also fabulous as a make-ahead breakfast for busy weekdays.

Yield: 8 servings

Prep Time: 15 minutes

Cook Time: 30 minutes

Total Time: 45 minutes

_____

NUT-FREE

- 4 cups (624 g) frozen broccoli, thawed and drained
- 10 ounces (280 g) chicken breakfast sausage, cooked and chopped (see Tips)
- 8 ounces (225 g) bacon, cooked crisp and crumbled
- 1 cup (180 g) chopped fresh tomatoes
- 8 large eggs
- ⅓ cup (80 ml) heavy whipping cream
- 4 garlic cloves, minced
- 1 teaspoon Italian seasoning
- ¾ teaspoon salt
- ½ teaspoon ground black pepper
- 1 cup (115 g) shredded cheddar cheese

1. Preheat the oven to 375°F (190°C or gas mark 5) and grease a glass or ceramic 9 × 13-inch (23 × 33 cm) pan.

2. Layer the broccoli, sausage, bacon, and tomatoes in the bottom of the pan.

3. In a large bowl, whisk the eggs, cream, garlic, Italian seasoning, salt, and pepper to blend. Pour the eggs over the ingredients in the pan. Sprinkle the top with the cheese.

4. Bake for 25 to 30 minutes until the top is golden brown and set in the middle. Let cool for at least 10 minutes before serving.

Tips

- If you only have fresh broccoli, cook it a little first so it softens properly. Steam it in a pot or in the microwave on high power for about 3 minutes until it's fork-tender.

- Use turkey, pork, or chicken breakfast sausage, according to your taste. I use chicken sausage, so the nutritional information is based on that.

- A glass or ceramic dish works best for this casserole, as it conducts heat more slowly than metal pans. Metal may cause the bottom and edges to get too dark.

Nutritional Information | Calories: 418 | Total Carbs: 5.7 g | Dietary Fiber: 1.5 g | Protein: 29.5 g | Fat: 27.3 g | Saturated Fat: 12.6 g

Garlic and Herb Scrambled Eggs

Cottage cheese adds flavor, creaminess, and protein to classic scrambled eggs. Add some garlic and a touch of dill for an easy, delicious breakfast. Pair this dish with some Turkey Breakfast Sausage (page 48) for a super-high-protein breakfast.

Yield: 4 servings

Prep Time: 5 minutes

Cook Time: 14 minutes

Total Time: 19 minutes

NUT-FREE, VEGETARIAN

1 tablespoon (15 ml) olive oil

8 large eggs

1 cup (225 g) cottage cheese

3 tablespoons (12 g) chopped fresh dill, plus more for garnish

2 garlic cloves, minced

½ teaspoon salt

½ teaspoon ground black pepper

1. Set a 12-inch (30 cm) nonstick skillet over medium-low heat and pour in the oil.

2. In a large bowl, whisk the eggs, cottage cheese, dill, garlic, salt, and pepper until well combined.

3. Pour the mixture into the pan and cook for 1 to 2 minutes, undisturbed, until the edges begin to set. Use a rubber spatula to scoop and fold the eggs from the outer edges of the pan toward the center. Continue to cook, scooping and folding every few minutes, until the eggs are set to your liking, 10 to 12 minutes.

4. Taste and adjust the seasonings. Serve with a sprinkle of chopped dill.

Tips

- If you prefer a smooth mixture without the curds, combine the eggs and cottage cheese in a blender for 30 seconds. Mix in the remaining ingredients by hand and proceed with step 2.

- If your skillet is not nonstick, you may need to use an additional tablespoon (15 ml) of oil.

Nutritional Information | Calories: 214 | Total Carbs: 2.8 g | Dietary Fiber: 0 g | Protein: 19.7 g | Fat: 13.2 g | Saturated Fat: 4.3 g

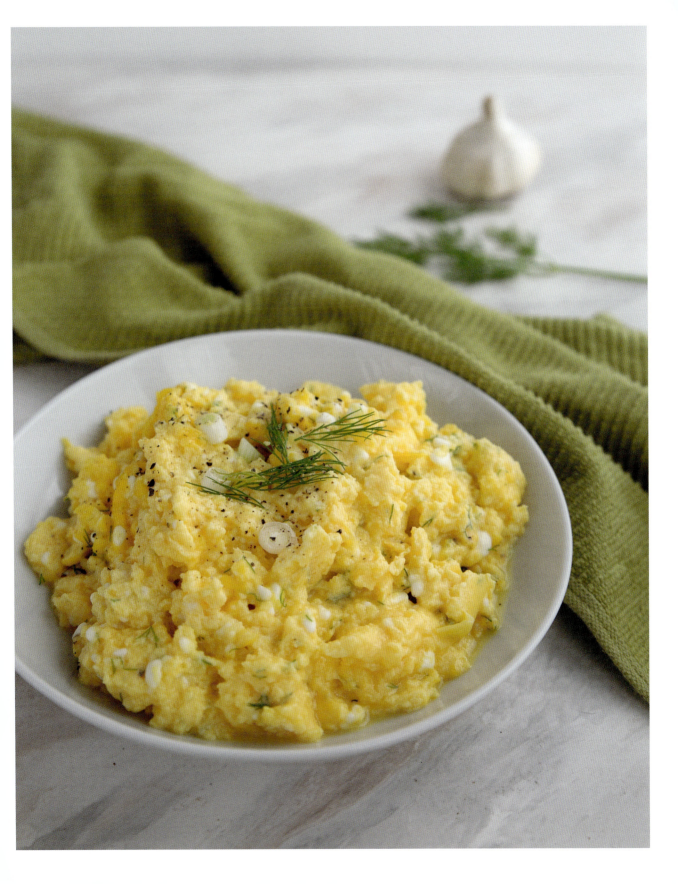

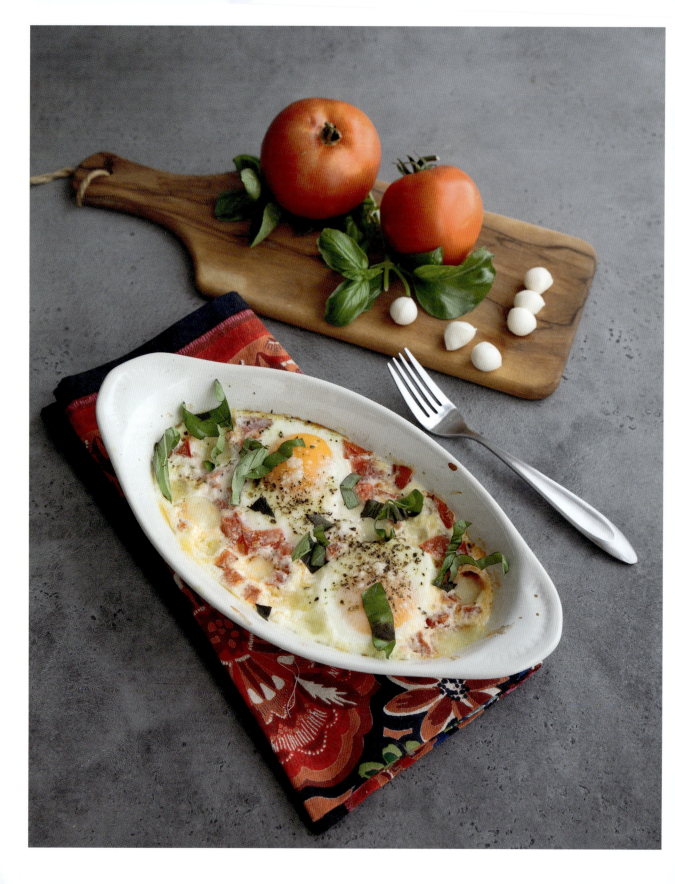

Caprese Baked Eggs

These Italian-style baked eggs have all the luscious flavor of Caprese salad in one easy breakfast dish. Make as many or as few servings as you need. Toast some Rustic Nut and Seed Bread (page 76) for dipping into the gooey egg yolks.

Yield: 2 servings

Prep Time: 15 minutes

Cook Time: 15 minutes

Total Time: 30 minutes

NUT-FREE, VEGETARIAN

2 teaspoons unsalted butter

4 large eggs

2 ounces (55 g) bocconcini (fresh raw mozzarella), chopped

1 small tomato, chopped

½ teaspoon salt

½ teaspoon Italian seasoning

¼ teaspoon ground black pepper

¼ ounce (7 g) grated parmesan cheese

1 tablespoon (3 g) fresh chopped basil

1. Preheat the oven to 375°F (190°C or gas mark 5).

2. Divide the butter between two 8-ounce (225 g) ramekins. Place the ramekins in the oven to melt the butter, then use a pastry brush to spread it all over the bottom and sides of the dishes.

3. Gently crack 2 eggs into each of the ramekins, keeping the yolks intact, or breaking them, if you prefer. Divide the bocconcini and tomato between the 2 ramekins, sprinkling them over and around the eggs. Sprinkle each with salt, Italian seasoning, pepper, and parmesan.

4. Bake for 12 to 15 minutes, or until the eggs are set to your liking. The whites should be completely set.

5. Top with fresh basil and serve hot.

Tips

- How long the eggs take to bake can depend on how deep your baking dishes are. Mine allow the eggs to spread a bit more than deeper ramekins do.

- You can also use a larger baking dish and make multiple servings in one dish. Scale up or down as needed!

Nutritional Information | Calories: 291 | Total Carbs: 5.2 g | Dietary Fiber: 1.1 g | Protein: 21 g | Fat: 19.1 g | Saturated Fat: 9.9 g

Make-Ahead Breakfast Bowls

These breakfast bowls are my healthy answer to the carb-laden breakfast bowls found in the freezer aisle of most grocery stores. They can be prepped ahead and frozen for when you need them.

Yield: 4 servings

Prep Time: 25 minutes

Cook Time: 20 minutes

Total Time: 45 minutes

NUT-FREE

- 2 tablespoons (28 ml) olive oil, divided
- 4 ounces (115 g) cremini or button mushrooms, sliced
- 1 medium-size zucchini, halved lengthwise and cut into ¼-inch (6 mm)-thick slices
- Salt and ground black pepper
- 8 ounces (225 g) frozen cauliflower florets, thawed
- 4 ounces (115 g) precooked breakfast sausage or Turkey Breakfast Sausage (page 48), sliced
- 8 large eggs
- 2 tablespoons (28 ml) heavy whipping cream
- 2 garlic cloves, minced
- 1 cup (115 g) shredded cheddar cheese

1. In a large skillet over medium heat, heat 1 tablespoon (15 ml) of the oil until hot. Add the mushrooms and zucchini and season generously with salt and pepper. Cook until the vegetables are tender and a little browned, 5 to 6 minutes.

2. Stir in the cauliflower florets to combine. Cook until warmed through, another 2 minutes. Divide both the vegetables and the sausage among 4 freezer-safe, microwave-safe containers.

3. In a large bowl, whisk the eggs, cream, and garlic until well combined.

4. Pour the remaining tablespoon (15 ml) oil into the skillet over medium-low heat.

5. Add the egg mixture and cook for 2 minutes, undisturbed, then use a rubber spatula to scrape the eggs from the edges of the pan toward the center. When the eggs are just cooked through, remove the pan from the heat and season to taste with salt and pepper. Divide the eggs among the containers. Sprinkle each with cheese.

6. Once at room temperature, cover and freeze for up to 2 weeks or refrigerate for up to 5 days.

Tips

- If you are using glass containers, let them sit out for 30 to 40 minutes before microwaving. A rapid change in temperature can shatter the glass.

Nutritional Information | Calories: 404 | Total Carbs: 7 g | Dietary Fiber: 2 g | Protein: 26.3 g | Fat: 28 g | Saturated Fat: 11.8 g

Breakfast Enchiladas

Try this low-carb twist on a breakfast favorite. Using slices of deli ham or turkey in place of the tortillas adds even more high-quality protein. It also makes a wonderful BFD (breakfast for dinner!). See top right of page 34 for photo.

Yield: 4 servings
(2 enchiladas per serving)

Prep Time: 20 minutes

Cook Time: 40 minutes

Total Time: 1 hour

NUT–FREE

FOR SAUCE:

1½ tablespoons (24 g) tomato paste

⅓ cup (80 ml) water

1 tablespoon (8 g) chili powder

½ teaspoon ground cumin

½ teaspoon salt

⅛ teaspoon cayenne pepper

FOR ENCHILADAS:

1 tablespoon (15 ml) avocado oil

8 large eggs

2 tablespoons (28 ml) heavy whipping cream

2 medium scallions, white and light green parts, thinly sliced, divided

2 garlic cloves, minced

½ teaspoon salt

½ teaspoon ground black pepper

8 slices uncured deli ham or turkey (about 1 ounce, or 28 g, each)

1 cup (115 g) shredded cheddar or Mexican cheese blend

1 tablespoon (1 g) chopped fresh cilantro

1. To make the sauce: In a medium bowl, whisk all of the sauce ingredients until smooth.

2. To make the enchiladas: Set a 12-inch (30 cm) skillet over medium-low heat and pour in the oil.

3. In a large bowl, whisk the eggs, cream, half of the scallions, garlic, salt, and black pepper until well combined. Pour the mixture into the pan and let cook for 1 to 2 minutes, undisturbed, until the edges begin to set. Use a rubber spatula to scoop and fold the eggs from the outer edges of the pan toward the center. Continue to cook, scooping and folding every few minutes, until the eggs are set to your liking, 10 to 12 minutes.

4. Preheat the oven to 350°F (180°C or gas mark 4) and grease a 1½- to 2-quart (1.4 to 1.9 L) glass or ceramic baking dish.

5. Lay the ham or turkey slices on a work surface. Spoon the scrambled eggs along the center of each and roll up tightly. Place the rolls in the prepared baking dish, seam-side down.

6. Drizzle the tops of the rolls with the enchilada sauce, then sprinkle the whole dish with the cheese.

7. Bake for 20 to 25 minutes until the cheese is melted and bubbly. Let cool for 5 minutes, then sprinkle with the remaining scallions and the cilantro.

Nutritional Information | Calories: 345 | Total Carbs: 5.5 g | Dietary Fiber: 1.1 g | Protein: 25.1 g | Fat: 23.9 g | Saturated Fat: 11 g

Spinach Mushroom Egg Muffins

Egg muffins are the ultimate grab-and-go protein breakfast. Make a big batch and enjoy them all week long. I make them jumbo-size, but they are just as good if made as standard-size muffins.

Yield: 5 servings (1 jumbo or 2 standard muffins per serving)

Prep Time: 20 minutes

Cook Time: 30 minutes

Total Time: 50 minutes

NUT-FREE, VEGETARIAN

2 tablespoons (28 ml) olive oil

6 ounces (170 g) mushrooms, halved and sliced

1 garlic clove, minced

8 ounces (225 g) chopped frozen spinach, thawed

8 large eggs

⅓ cup (80 ml) heavy whipping cream

¼ cup (28 g) coconut flour

½ ounce (14 g) freshly grated parmesan cheese

1 teaspoon baking powder

¾ teaspoon salt

½ teaspoon ground black pepper

¼ teaspoon red pepper flakes (optional)

1. Preheat the oven to 375°F (190°C or gas mark 5) and line a jumbo muffin tin with 5 jumbo silicone or parchment paper liners. Alternatively, line a standard muffin tin with 10 silicone or parchment liners.

2. In a medium skillet over medium heat, heat the oil until hot. Add the mushrooms and sauté until golden, 4 to 5 minutes. Add the garlic and sauté for 1 minute.

3. Squeeze the chopped spinach to release any excess moisture and add the spinach to the mushrooms, breaking up any clumps with a wooden spoon.

4. In a large bowl, whisk the eggs, cream, coconut flour, parmesan, baking powder, salt, black pepper, and red pepper flakes (if using) until well combined. Stir in the mushroom-spinach mixture until well distributed. Divide the batter evenly among the prepared muffin cups.

5. Bake for 25 to 30 minutes, or until set and just firm to the touch. If making smaller muffins, bake for 20 to 25 minutes. Let cool for at least 10 minutes before serving. Store in an airtight container in the refrigerator for up to 5 days or in the freezer for 2 months.

Tips

- Using coconut flour and baking powder gives these muffins a little structure so they don't rise and then collapse into themselves. It also adds fiber, making them even more satisfying.

- When baking low-carb muffins and cupcakes, always use parchment or silicone liners. Paper liners stick badly, and you will lose too much of your precious muffin.

Nutritional Information | Calories: 262 | Total Carbs: 8.1 g | Dietary Fiber: 3.5 g | Protein: 13.7 g | Fat: 18.6 g | Saturated Fat: 7.7 g

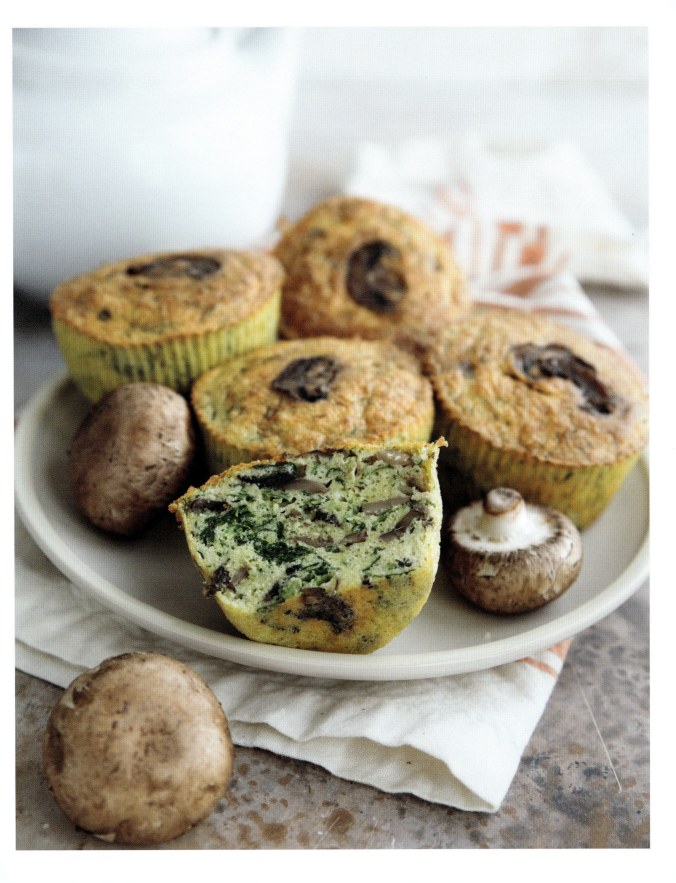

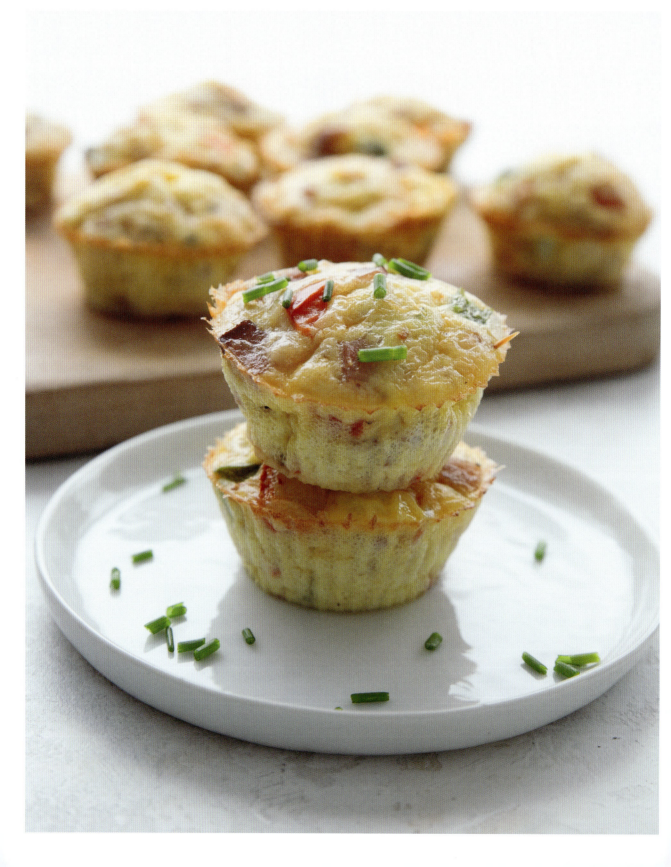

Denver Omelet Cups

Packed with protein, these easy Denver omelet cups offer a fabulous low-carb, high-protein breakfast option. They freeze well too so you can sock them away for busy weekday mornings.

Yield: 6 servings (2 omelet cups per serving)

Prep Time: 15 minutes

Cook Time: 40 minutes

Total Time: 55 minutes

NUT-FREE

2 tablespoons (28 g) unsalted butter

8 ounces (225 g) diced ham

½ medium-size red bell pepper, finely chopped

½ medium-size green bell pepper, finely chopped

¼ cup (40 g) diced onion

6 large eggs

¼ cup (60 ml) heavy whipping cream

½ teaspoon salt

¼ teaspoon ground black pepper

1 cup (115 g) shredded cheddar cheese

1. Preheat the oven to 350°F (180°C or gas mark 4) and line a standard muffin tin with 12 silicone or parchment paper liners.

2. In a large skillet over medium heat, melt the butter. Once hot, add the ham and sauté until browned and crispy, about 2 minutes.

3. Add the bell peppers and onion and continue to cook, stirring frequently, until tender, about 4 minutes more. Let cool for at least 15 minutes.

4. In a large bowl, whisk the eggs, cream, salt, and pepper to blend. Stir in the ham-vegetable mixture, then stir in the cheese. Divide the mixture among the prepared muffin cups.

5. Bake for about 30 minutes until puffed and golden brown. Let cool for at least 10 minutes before serving.

Tips

If you freeze these, wrap them tightly in plastic wrap to avoid freezer burn. Thaw them completely before rewarming gently in the oven or microwave.

Nutritional Information | Calories: 285 | Total Carbs: 4.1 g | Dietary Fiber: 1 g | Protein: 17.6 g | Fat: 20 g | Saturated Fat: 11.1 g

Turkey Breakfast Sausage

Making your own breakfast sausage is easier than you think and far healthier too. There's no added sugars or preservatives. Freeze and reheat as needed.

Yield: 4 servings (2 patties per serving)

Prep Time: 15 minutes

Cook Time: 10 minutes per batch

Total Time: 25 minutes

DAIRY-FREE, EGG-FREE, NUT-FREE

- 1 pound (455 g) ground turkey
- 2 garlic cloves, minced
- 1 tablespoon (3 g) chopped fresh sage
- 1 teaspoon salt
- ¾ teaspoon coarsely ground black pepper
- ¾ teaspoon fennel seeds, crushed
- ½ teaspoon red pepper flakes
- ½ teaspoon paprika
- 2 tablespoons (28 ml) avocado or olive oil

1. Line a plate with wax paper.

2. In a large bowl, combine the ground turkey, garlic, sage, salt, black pepper, fennel seeds, red pepper flakes, and paprika. Use your hands to mix all the ingredients well. Form the mixture into 8 small, flat patties and place on the prepared plate.

3. In a large skillet over medium heat, heat the oil until it shimmers. Cook the patties, in batches as needed, for 4 to 5 minutes per side until the centers reach 165°F (74°C) on an instant-read thermometer.

Tips

Freeze the sausage patties cooked or uncooked. If they are uncooked, set them in the freezer on the wax paper–lined plate until completely frozen, then store them in a freezer-safe container. Thaw completely before cooking.

Nutritional Information | Calories: 207 | Total Carbs: 1 g | Dietary Fiber: 0.3 g | Protein: 21.5 g | Fat: 15.6 g | Saturated Fat: 3.5 g

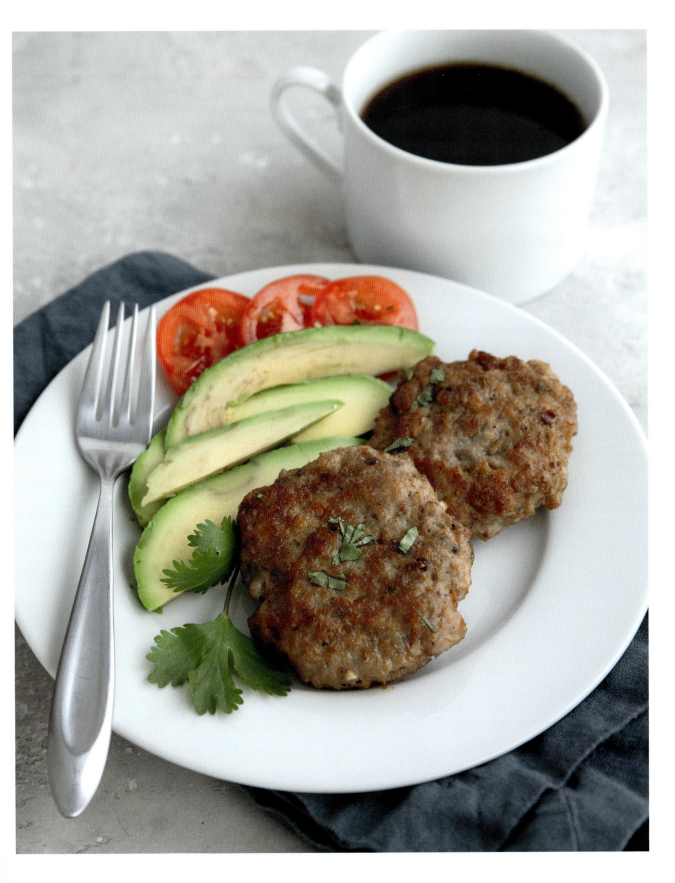

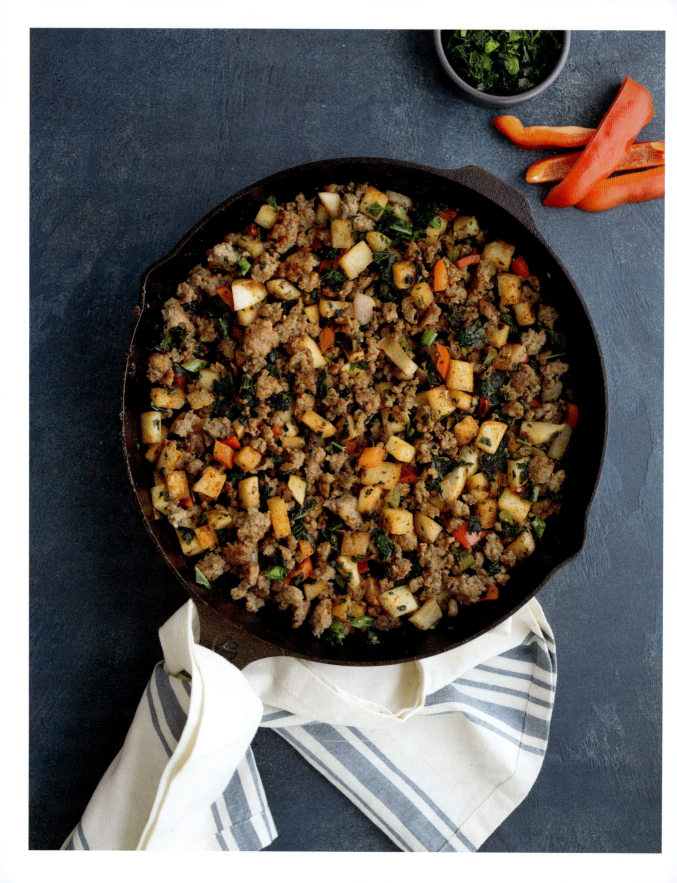

Sausage Breakfast Hash

Classic breakfast hash gets a low-carb, high-protein makeover. Turnips are a delicious replacement for potatoes. And while I designed this recipe to be egg-free, you can always throw a fried egg on top for added protein.

Yield: 4 servings

Prep Time: 10 minutes

Cook Time: 25 minutes

Total Time: 35 minutes

DAIRY-FREE, EGG-FREE, NUT-FREE

- 1¼ pounds (570 g) bulk breakfast sausage
- 1 tablespoon (15 ml) olive oil
- 2 medium-size turnips, diced
- ¼ cup (40 g) chopped onion
- ¾ teaspoon salt
- ½ teaspoon ground black pepper
- ½ medium-size red bell pepper, chopped
- 6 ounces (170 g) frozen kale, thawed and drained
- ½ teaspoon garlic powder
- ½ teaspoon smoked paprika
- ¼ teaspoon red pepper flakes (optional)

1. In a large skillet over medium heat, cook the breakfast sausage, breaking it up with a wooden spoon, until browned and cooked through, about 8 minutes. Use a slotted spoon to transfer the sausage to a bowl, leaving any drippings behind.

2. Pour the oil into the skillet. Once hot, add the turnips and onion and toss to coat. Season with the salt and black pepper and cook, stirring frequently, until the turnips become tender, about 8 minutes.

3. Stir in the red bell pepper, kale, garlic powder, paprika, and red pepper flakes (if using) and cook for 3 to 4 minutes until just tender.

4. Return the sausage to the pan and stir to combine and warm through. Serve hot.

Tips

- Dice the turnip as evenly as possible into ½-inch (1 cm) cubes, so they cook more quickly.

- Substitute other sausages here. Try hot or mild Italian, or turkey or chicken sausage, which will be slightly higher in protein.

Nutritional Information | Calories: 379 | Total Carbs: 7.7 g | Dietary Fiber: 2.4 g | Protein: 23.9 g | Fat: 25.6 g | Saturated Fat: 9.5 g

Easy Baked Pancakes

Don't feel like standing there flipping pancakes over a hot skillet? Try my easy oven-baked method. Top the pancakes with chocolate chips or berries or just leave them plain. They are also delicious with a smear of peanut butter or my high-protein Chocolate Hazelnut Spread (page 121).

Yield: 4 servings

Prep Time: 10 minutes

Cook Time: 15 minutes

Total Time: 25 minutes

NUT-FREE OPTION, VEGETARIAN

½ cup (120 g) high-protein yogurt

4 large eggs

2 tablespoons (28 ml) avocado oil

1 teaspoon vanilla extract

½ cup (60 g) plain or vanilla whey protein powder

½ cup (56 g) almond flour, or 3 tablespoons (21 g) coconut flour (nut-free option)

¼ cup (48 g) granular sweetener

1 teaspoon baking powder

¼ teaspoon salt

2 tablespoons (30 g) sugar-free chocolate chips

1. Preheat the oven to 350°F (180°C or gas mark 4) and grease an 8 × 8-inch (20 × 20 cm) ceramic baking dish.

2. In a blender, combine the yogurt, eggs, oil, and vanilla. Blend until well combined.

3. Add the protein powder, almond flour, sweetener, baking powder, and salt and blend again until smooth. Let the batter rest for 5 minutes.

4. Pour the batter into the prepared baking dish and sprinkle the top with the chocolate chips.

5. Bake for 12 to 15 minutes, or until puffed and just firm to the touch. Let cool for 5 minutes before serving.

Tips

- I do not recommend using egg white protein for this recipe, as the results will be very rubbery.

- If you don't have a glass or ceramic baking dish, line a metal pan with parchment paper and grease the parchment. The baking time may change a little, so keep an eye on the pancake while it is in the oven.

Nutritional Information | Calories: 278 | Total Carbs: 7.9 g | Dietary Fiber: 3.5 g | Protein: 23.4 g | Fat: 21.2 g | Saturated Fat: 4.8 g

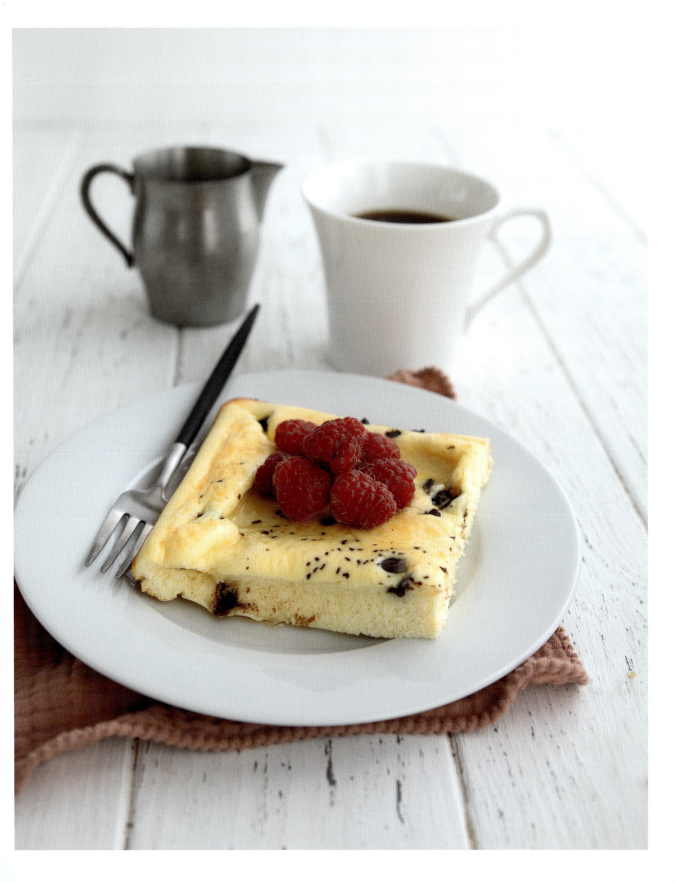

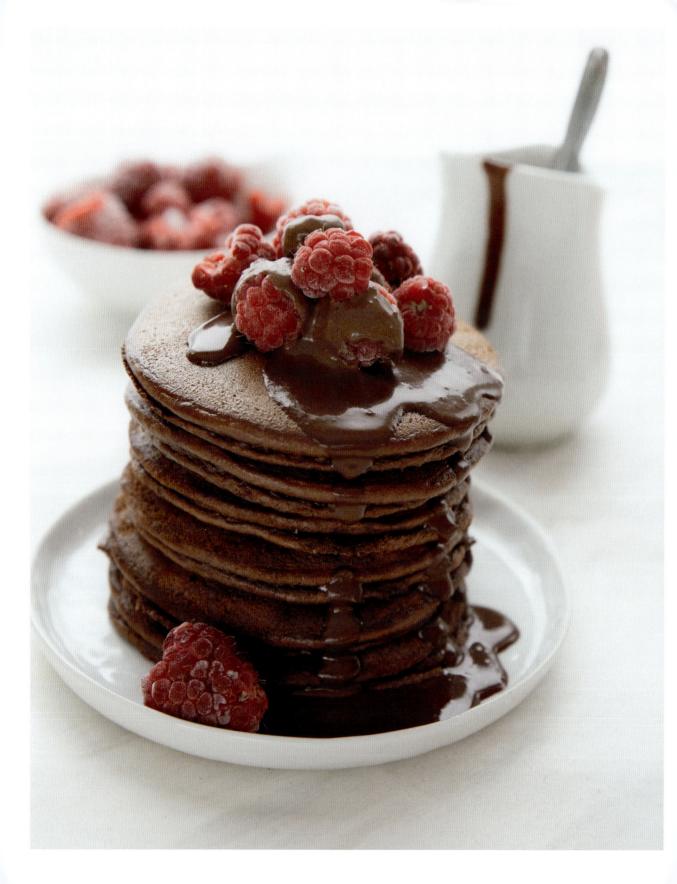

Chocolate Protein Pancakes

Who doesn't want to start their day with chocolate? Especially when it's high protein and low carb.

Yield: Makes 18 small pancakes (3 pancakes per serving)

Prep Time: 5 minutes

Cook Time: 25 minutes

Total Time: 30 minutes

NUT-FREE OPTION, VEGETARIAN

4 ounces (115 g) cream cheese, softened

3 large eggs

¼ cup (60 ml) unsweetened almond or hemp milk (nut-free option)

1 teaspoon vanilla extract

1 cup (110 g) pumpkin seed meal

¾ cup (72 g) chocolate protein powder

⅓ cup (64 g) granular sweetener

2 teaspoons baking powder

1 tablespoon (5 g) cocoa powder

Avocado oil, for cooking

1. In a large blender, combine the cream cheese, eggs, almond milk, and vanilla. Blend until smooth.

2. Add the pumpkin seed meal, protein powder, sweetener, baking powder, and cocoa powder and blend again until well combined and smooth.

3. Heat a large nonstick skillet or griddle over medium heat and lightly grease it with a little oil. Use about 3 tablespoons (45 ml) of the batter for each pancake, working in batches as needed. Cook until bubbles begin to appear on the tops of the pancakes and the edges are set and dry, 3 to 4 minutes. Carefully wiggle a thin-blade spatula under the pancakes and flip them over. Continue to cook until the second side is nicely browned, 3 or 4 minutes. Repeat with the remaining batter, adding more oil to the pan as needed.

Tips

- If you can't find or make pumpkin seed meal, use almond flour or another nut or seed flour.

- Keep the pancakes on the small side so they are easier to flip.

Protein powder options

I recommend whey, egg white, or vegan protein powders. If you don't have chocolate protein powder, add an additional tablespoon (5 g) of cocoa powder. You may need a little more liquid in the batter.

Nutritional Information | Calories: 265 | Total Carbs: 6.8 g | Dietary Fiber: 1.4 g | Protein: 19.7 g | Fat: 16.7 g | Saturated Fat: 6.5 g

Cottage Cheese Waffles

Cottage cheese is both high in protein and incredibly versatile, which is why you see it in so many high-protein recipes. Turns out it's great in waffles too.

Yield: 6 servings (serving size depends on your waffle iron)

Prep Time: 10 minutes

Cook Time: 20 minutes

Total Time: 30 minutes

VEGETARIAN

⅔ cup (150 g) cottage cheese

3 large eggs, at room temperature

1 teaspoon vanilla extract

⅔ cup (75 g) almond flour

½ cup (60 g) unflavored whey protein powder

¼ cup (48 g) granular sweetener

1 teaspoon baking powder

¼ teaspoon salt

3 tablespoons (45 ml) melted unsalted butter or avocado oil

1. In a blender, combine the cottage cheese, eggs, and vanilla. Blend until smooth.

2. Add the almond flour, protein powder, sweetener, baking powder, and salt and blend again until smooth.

3. With the blender running on low speed, pour the melted butter into the mixture until well combined.

4. Meanwhile, preheat the waffle iron according to the manufacturer's instructions and grease it lightly.

5. For mini waffles, add about ¼ cup (60 ml) of the batter to the iron. For classic round waffles, you will need more like ⅓ cup (80 ml). Close the lid and cook until puffed and golden brown. The time will vary depending on your waffle iron. Remove the waffles and repeat with the remaining batter.

Tips

- If using a mini waffle iron, you'll get about 12 waffles (2 per serving). For a classic round waffle maker, you'll get about 6 waffles. Deep Belgian-style waffle makers will take more batter per section, so you'll get fewer waffles.

- I recommend an erythritol-based sweetener if you want a crisper texture. Allulose will cause the waffles to brown quite a bit more, preventing them from crisping.

Protein powder options

Whey protein is the best option for these waffles, although some vegan proteins may work as well. Egg white protein makes the waffles very rubbery!

Nutritional Information | Calories: 209 | Total Carbs: 4.5 g | Dietary Fiber: 1.3 g | Protein: 16.7 g | Fat: 14.6 g | Saturated Fat: 5.5 g

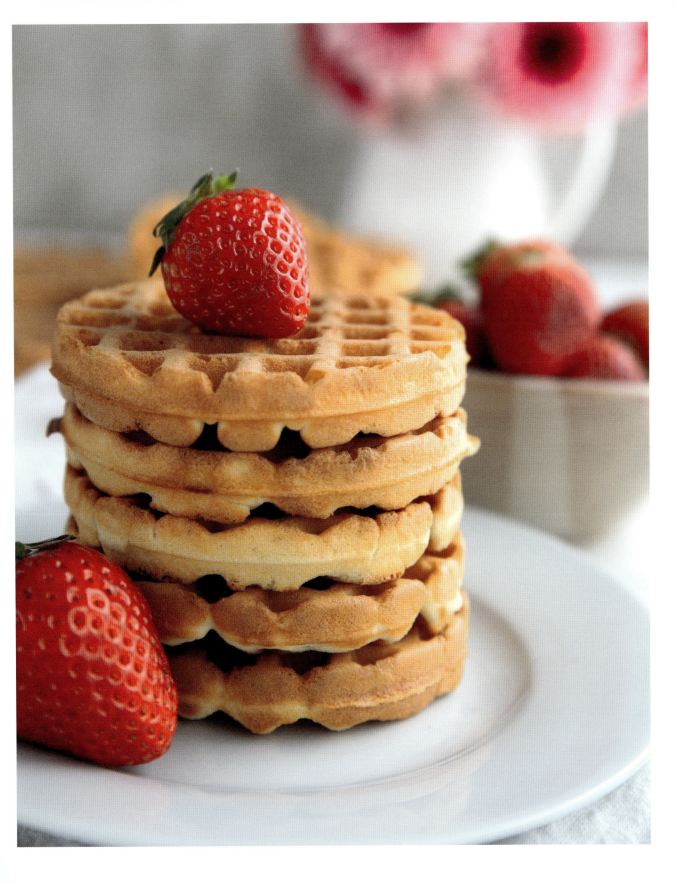

Cheddar Zucchini Waffles

These crispy, savory keto waffles are packed with sharp cheddar and zucchini. Easy to make and grain-free, they make great sandwiches too.

Yield: 6 servings (serving size depends on your waffle iron)

Prep Time: 1 hour 10 minutes (includes 1 hour to drain)

Cook Time: 20 minutes

Total Time: 1 hour 30 minutes

VEGETARIAN

1 medium-size zucchini, grated

½ teaspoon salt, divided

4 large eggs

6 ounces (170 g) shredded sharp cheddar cheese

1 garlic clove, minced

¼ teaspoon ground black pepper

¼ teaspoon cayenne pepper

¾ cup (84 g) almond flour

2 teaspoons baking powder

3 tablespoons (45 ml) heavy whipping cream

1. Place the zucchini in a sieve in the sink or set over a bowl and sprinkle with ¼ teaspoon of the salt. Toss to combine and let drain for 1 hour. Squeeze out as much moisture as possible.

2. Preheat the waffle iron according to the manufacturer's instructions and lightly grease it with butter or oil.

3. In a large bowl, whisk the eggs to break them up. Whisk in the cheese, zucchini, garlic, remaining ¼ teaspoon salt, black pepper, and cayenne until well combined. Add the almond flour and baking powder and stir to combine, then stir in the cream.

4. For mini waffles, add about 3 tablespoons (45 ml) of the batter to the iron. For classic round waffles, you will need more like ¼ cup (60 ml). Close the lid and cook until golden brown and crispy. The time will vary depending on your waffle iron. Remove the waffles and repeat with the remaining batter.

Tips

- If using a mini waffle iron, you will get about 12 waffles (2 per serving). For a classic round waffle maker, you will get about 6 waffles. Deep Belgian-style waffle makers will take more batter per section, so you will get fewer waffles.

- These savory waffles are sturdy enough to be used as bread, and they make great breakfast sandwiches. I love making them as mini waffles for this reason!

Nutritional Information | Calories: 275 | Total Carbs: 5.5 g | Dietary Fiber: 1.9 g | Protein: 14.6 g | Fat: 20.1 g | Saturated Fat: 8.8 g

Peanut Butter Granola

I have a popular low-carb granola recipe on my website that readers love. And I was delighted to discover that, with a few tweaks here and there, I could turn it into a high-protein treat that's great for easy breakfasts and snacks.

Yield: 10 servings (about ⅓ cup, or 50 g, per serving)

Prep Time: 15 minutes

Cook Time: 30 minutes

Total Time: 45 minutes

DAIRY-FREE OPTION, EGG-FREE, VEGETARIAN

1 cup (136 g) shelled pumpkin seeds

¾ cup (83 g) chopped pecans

½ cup (80 g) hemp seeds

⅓ cup (20 g) unsweetened flaked coconut

½ cup (60 g) plain or vanilla whey protein powder

¼ cup (48 g) erythritol sweetener

½ teaspoon salt

⅓ cup (87 g) creamy peanut butter

4 tablespoons (55 g) unsalted butter, plus more as needed

½ teaspoon vanilla extract

Protein powder options

I recommend whey, egg white, or hemp seed protein for this recipe. Do not use collagen or bone broth protein, as it won't crisp up properly.

1. Preheat the oven to 300°F (150°C or gas mark 2) and line a large, rimmed baking sheet with parchment paper.

2. In a food processor, combine the pumpkin seeds, pecans, hemp seeds, and coconut. Pulse a few times until the mixture resembles coarse crumbs with some larger pieces. Transfer to a large bowl and stir in the protein powder, sweetener, and salt.

3. In a microwave-safe bowl, melt together the peanut butter and butter on high power for 30 to 60 seconds. Stir in the vanilla. Pour the mixture over the granola and stir until it begins to clump. If the mixture is dry, stir in an additional tablespoon (15 ml) of melted butter. Spread the granola evenly on the prepared baking sheet and press it down firmly with a flat-bottomed glass.

4. Bake for 30 minutes, stirring halfway through and re-pressing it down. Let cool completely, then break up any large clumps with your hands. Store in an airtight container at room temperature for up to 1 week.

Tips

- I specify erythritol for this recipe because any amount of allulose or xylitol will keep the granola from crisping up properly. Add some additional sweetness with stevia or monk fruit extract, if you like.

- For a dairy-free granola, use melted coconut oil in place of the butter and choose egg white or hemp protein powder.

Nutritional Information | Calories: 289 | Total Carbs: 6.6 g | Dietary Fiber: 3.1 g | Protein: 13.3 g | Fat: 23.9 g | Saturated Fat: 6 g

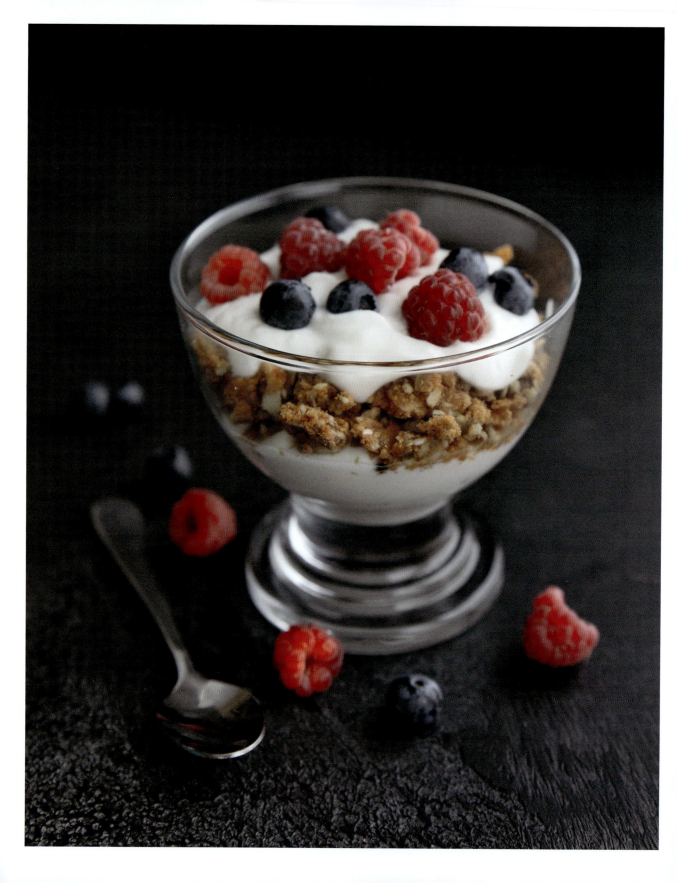

Yogurt Granola Parfait

Yogurt and granola make a classic breakfast combo, but it's usually full of sugar. Well, no longer! With 28 grams of protein, this easy breakfast will fuel you through your morning.

Yield: 1 serving

Prep Time: 5 minutes

Total Time: 5 minutes

_____

EGG-FREE, VEGETARIAN

½ cup (120 g) high-protein yogurt

2 tablespoons (15 g) whey protein powder

2 teaspoons powdered sweetener

¼ teaspoon vanilla extract

3 tablespoons (30 g) Peanut Butter Granola (page 59)

Fresh berries, for serving

1. In a small bowl, whisk the yogurt, protein powder, sweetener, and vanilla to blend.

2. Sprinkle about half of the granola into a small glass dessert dish. Spoon half of the yogurt mixture over the granola. Repeat the layers.

3. Top with the berries to serve.

Tips

If you use flavored protein powder and/or yogurt, you may not need the sweetener or the vanilla extract.

Nutritional Information (not including berries) | Calories: 268 | Total Carbs: 7 g | Dietary Fiber: 1.8 g | Protein: 28.1 g | Fat: 15.5 g | Saturated Fat: 3.9 g

Hot Maple Cereal

This low-carb hot breakfast cereal couldn't be easier to make. Just heat up some water and you're ready to go. It's incredibly filling, just like the hot cereal you used to love. And because chia seeds and flaxseed contain tryptophan, this recipe offers a complete amino acid profile.

Yield: 2 servings (about ½ cup, or 90 g, per serving)

Prep Time: 5 minutes

Cook Time: 5 minutes

Total Time: 10 minutes

DAIRY-FREE, EGG-FREE, NUT-FREE

- ¼ cup (28 g) collagen protein powder
- 2 tablespoons (24 g) chia seeds
- 2 tablespoons (14 g) flaxseed meal
- 2 tablespoons (14 g) coconut flour
- Pinch salt
- ⅔ cup (160 ml) boiling water
- ½ teaspoon maple extract
- Sweetener, heavy whipping cream, or fresh berries, for serving

1. In a medium bowl, whisk the protein powder, chia seeds, flaxseed meal, coconut flour, and salt.

2. Add the water and stir until well combined. Let sit for 5 minutes to thicken, then stir in the maple extract.

3. Add sweetener to taste, divide between 2 bowls, and top as desired.

Tips

- You can use a flavored protein powder, but obviously that will add flavor to the porridge. If the protein powder is sweetened, you may not want any additional sweetener. You can also use vanilla extract in place of the maple extract.

- If you don't need to be nut-free, nut butter would also make a tasty topping.

Protein powder options

Collagen provides a thickness similar to classic hot porridge, but any protein powder should work.

Nutritional Information | Calories: 228 | Total Carbs: 11 g | Dietary Fiber: 9.4 g | Protein: 29.7 g | Fat: 8.3 g | Saturated Fat: 1.8 g

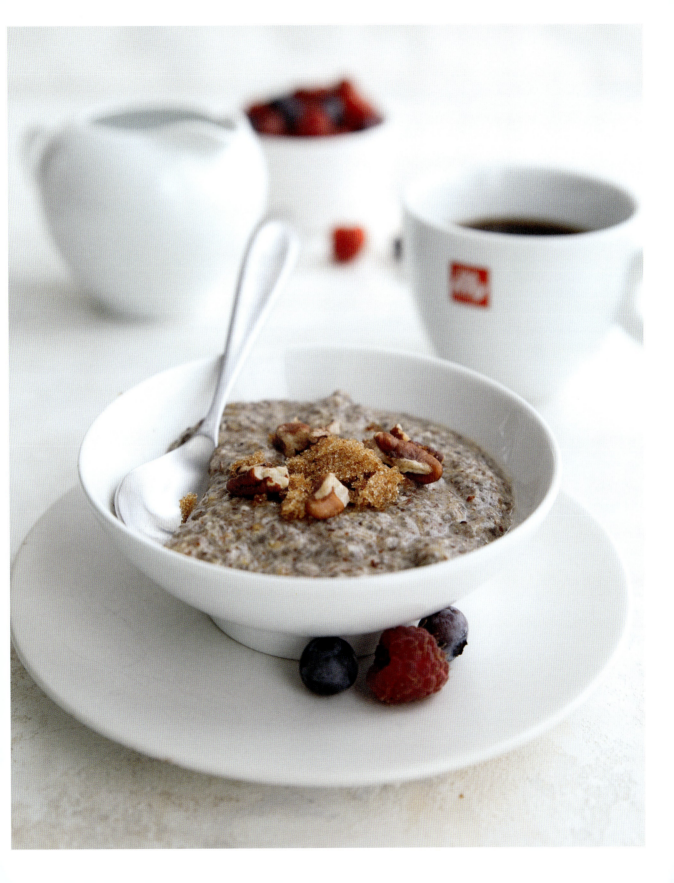

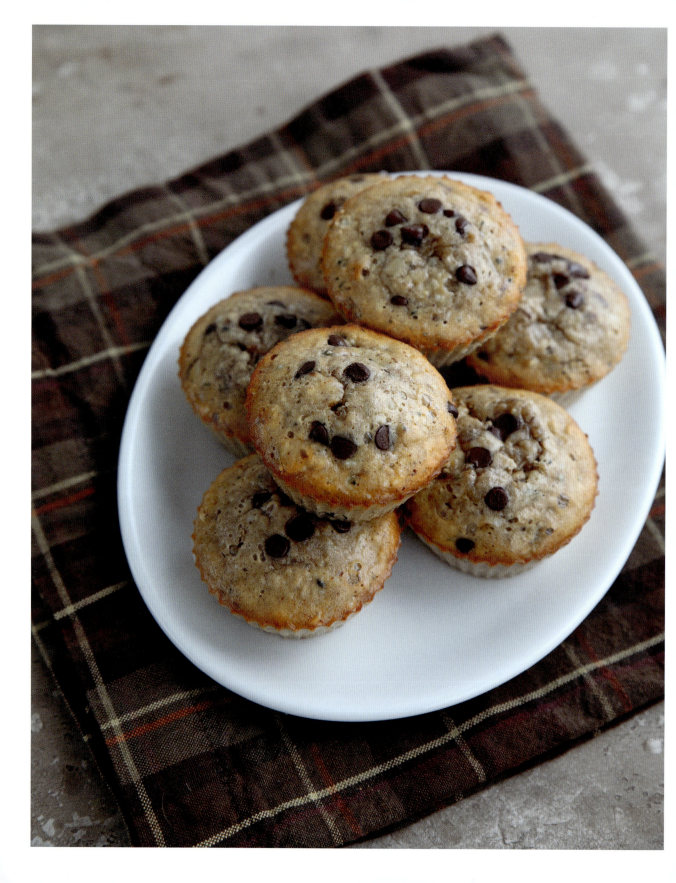

Baked Oatmeal Cups

This low-carb "faux oatmeal" contains no real oats. And baking it into cups makes it a perfect "grab-n-go" breakfast treat or easy snack.

Yield: 12 servings (1 oatmeal cup per serving)

Prep Time: 15 minutes

Cook Time: 25 minutes

Total Time: 40 minutes

1 cup (60 g) unsweetened flaked coconut

¾ cup (74 g) sliced almonds

½ cup (80 g) hemp seeds

⅓ cup (80 ml) avocado oil

⅓ cup (87 g) almond butter

½ cup (96 g) granular sweetener

2 large eggs, at room temperature

1 teaspoon vanilla extract

¾ cup (90 g) unflavored whey protein powder

¼ cup (28 g) collagen protein powder

½ teaspoon ground cinnamon

½ teaspoon salt

⅓ cup (80 g) sugar-free chocolate chips (optional)

1. Preheat the oven to 325°F (170°C or gas mark 3) and line a standard muffin tin with 12 silicone or parchment paper liners.

2. In a food processor, combine the coconut, almonds, and hemp seeds. Pulse until the mixture resembles oatmeal flakes. Set aside.

3. In a large bowl, whisk the oil, almond butter, and sweetener until well combined. Add the eggs and vanilla and whisk until smooth.

4. Add the coconut-almond mixture, protein powders, cinnamon, and salt and stir until well combined. Stir in the chocolate chips (if using). Divide the mixture among the prepared muffin cups, filling each about two-thirds full.

5. Bake for 20 to 25 minutes, or until the cups are slightly risen and set around the edges. They should still look a little wet in the center. Let cool in the pan.

Tips

- I like to make this recipe with a mix of allulose and erythritol sweeteners as I find it keeps the oatmeal cups a bit softer, like real oatmeal, but any sweetener will do.

- Some collagen also helps give them the right texture and helps keep them from drying out.

Nutritional Information | Calories: 264 | Total Carbs: 8.3 g | Dietary Fiber: 4.8 g | Protein: 16.6 g | Fat: 22.3 g | Saturated Fat: 3.7 g

Everything Bagel Smoked Salmon Toast

Yield: 1 serving

Prep Time: 5 minutes (not including bread baking time)

Total Time: 5 minutes

Sometimes a quick piece of toast is the ultimate convenience food. Keep a loaf of my Rustic Nut and Seed Bread (page 76) in the refrigerator to make this super healthy, protein-packed breakfast.

1 slice Rustic Nut and Seed Bread (page 76)

¼ cup (56 g) cottage cheese

2 ounces (55 g) lox-style smoked salmon

1½ teaspoons chopped red onion

1 teaspoon capers (optional)

¼ teaspoon everything bagel seasoning

1. Toast the bread.

2. Spread the toast with the cottage cheese and top with the smoked salmon, onion, capers (if using), and everything bagel seasoning.

Tips

Cottage cheese toast can have many variations. Whisk a little sweetener into the cottage cheese and add a few raspberries instead of salmon!

Nutritional Information | Calories: 279 | Total Carbs: 8.2 g | Dietary Fiber: 2.9 g | Protein: 26.5 g | Fat: 15.6 g | Saturated Fat: 3.3 g

Cinnamon Roll Breakfast Shake

This delicious protein smoothie is thick and frothy thanks to a rather unusual ingredient. Trust me, it works! See bottom left of page 34 for photo.

Yield: 1 smoothie

Prep Time: 5 minutes

Total Time: 5 minutes

EGG-FREE, NUT-FREE OPTION, VEGETARIAN

⅓ cup (80 g) high-protein yogurt

¼ cup (60 ml) unsweetened almond milk or hemp milk (nut-free option)

¼ cup (30 g) protein powder

½ teaspoon ground cinnamon, plus more as needed and for dusting

½ cup (43 g) frozen cauliflower florets, slightly thawed

½ cup (109 g) crushed ice

¼ teaspoon vanilla extract

Cinnamon, for serving

1. In a blender, combine all the ingredients and blend until smooth. Taste and adjust the sweetener and cinnamon. Pour into a glass and dust the top lightly with cinnamon before serving.

Tips

- Don't use frozen cauliflower rice, as the grains are so small they won't catch in the blender and your shake will end up grainy.

- If you use flavored yogurt or protein powder, you may not need any sweetener. You may also not need the vanilla extract.

Protein powder options

Use any protein you like best, but keep in mind that some may not provide a complete amino acid profile.

Nutritional Information | Calories: 236 | Total Carbs: 8.5 g | Dietary Fiber: 2.2 g | Protein: 34.3 g | Fat: 8.7 g | Saturated Fat: 4.5 g

Blueberry Breakfast Cake

I love a good coffee cake with a buttery streusel topping, and this high-protein version does not disappoint.

Yield: 10 servings
(1 slice per serving)

Prep Time: 20 minutes

Cook Time: 55 minutes

Total Time: 1 hour 15 minutes

VEGETARIAN

FOR CRUMB TOPPING:

¼ cup (28 g) finely chopped pecans

3 tablespoons (21 g) almond flour

3 tablespoons (36 g) brown sugar substitute

1 tablespoon (7 g) coconut flour

2 tablespoons (28 g) salted butter, melted

FOR CAKE:

½ cup (115 g) sour cream

2 large eggs

1 teaspoon vanilla extract

½ cup (96 g) granular sweetener

1¾ cups (196 g) almond flour

¾ cup (90 g) unflavored whey protein powder

2 teaspoons baking powder

½ teaspoon ground cinnamon

½ teaspoon salt

Water, as needed

¾ cup (109 g) fresh blueberries, divided

Powdered sweetener, for dusting (optional)

1. To make the crumb topping: In a medium bowl, whisk the pecans, almond flour, brown sugar substitute, and coconut flour to combine. Stir in the melted butter until the mixture resembles coarse crumbs.

2. Preheat the oven to 325°F (170°C or gas mark 3) and grease an 8-inch (20 cm) round cake pan. Line the bottom with parchment paper and grease the parchment.

3. To make the cake: In a large bowl, whisk the sour cream, eggs, vanilla, and granular sweetener to blend. Stir in the almond flour, protein powder, baking powder, cinnamon, and salt. If the batter is very thick, stir in water, 1 tablespoon (15 ml) at a time; it should be thick but easily spreadable.

4. Stir in ½ cup (73 g) of the blueberries, then spread the batter in the prepared baking pan. Scatter the remaining ¼ cup (36 g) berries on top, then sprinkle with the crumb topping.

5. Bake for 45 to 55 minutes until the top of the cake is just barely firm to the touch. Let cool completely in the pan, then run a sharp knife around the edges to loosen. Flip the cake onto a cake plate and dust with powdered sweetener (if using).

Tips

- I like using a brown sugar substitute for the topping, as it gives it a real streusel flavor, but any granular sweetener should work.

Nutritional Information | Calories: 251 | Total Carbs: 8.7 g | Dietary Fiber: 3.3 g | Protein: 13.7 g | Fat: 19.2 g | Saturated Fat: 4.9 g

- If you have a pan with a removable bottom, it makes it even easier to get this cake out without disturbing the topping!

Protein powder options

Whey or egg white protein powder works best in this recipe.

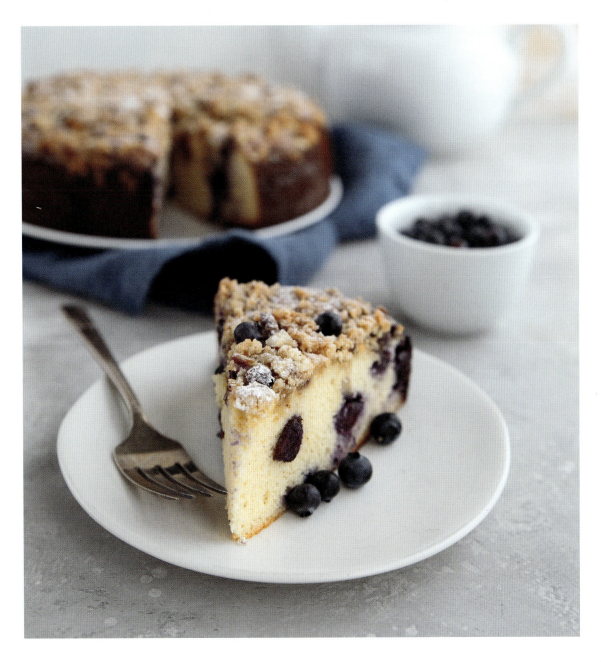

Zucchini Bread Breakfast Cookies

Who doesn't want to eat cookies for breakfast? Especially when they taste like zucchini bread and have almost 14 grams of protein per serving! See bottom right of page 34 for photo.

Yield: 8 cookies
(1 cookie per serving)

Prep Time: 1 hour 15 minutes
(includes 1 hour to drain)

Cook Time: 12 minutes

Total Time: 1 hour 27 minutes

DAIRY-FREE, EGG-FREE, VEGETARIAN

¾ cup (90 g) packed finely grated zucchini

¼ teaspoon salt

1 tablespoon (7 g) flaxseed meal

2 tablespoons (28 ml) water

½ cup (130 g) almond butter

1 tablespoon (15 ml) avocado oil

⅓ cup (64 g) brown sugar substitute

1 teaspoon vanilla extract

⅔ cup (72 g) vegan protein powder

3 tablespoons (30 g) hemp seeds

1½ teaspoons ground cinnamon

½ teaspoon grated nutmeg

½ teaspoon baking powder

¼ cup (30 g) chopped walnuts or (28 g) pecans (optional)

¼ cup (60 g) sugar-free chocolate chips (optional)

1. In a sieve over a bowl, combine the zucchini and salt. Let drain for 1 hour, then squeeze out as much moisture as possible.

2. Preheat the oven to 325°F (170°C or gas mark 3) and line a large baking sheet with a silicone mat or parchment paper. Lightly grease the mat or parchment.

3. In a small bowl, whisk the flaxseed meal and water to combine. Let sit for a few minutes to thicken.

4. In a large bowl, using a handheld electric mixer, beat together the almond butter, oil, and brown sugar substitute on medium speed. Beat in the zucchini, vanilla, and the flaxseed mixture.

5. Add the protein powder, hemp seeds, cinnamon, nutmeg, and baking powder and stir by hand until well combined. Spoon the dough into 8 mounds onto the prepared baking sheet. Without pressing down, use wet hands to shape them into rounds.

6. If using, top each cookie with nuts and chocolate chips.

7. Bake for 10 to 12 minutes until still soft to the touch but no longer sticky. Let cool completely on the pan.

Tips

This recipe works best with vegan protein. If using whey protein, the cookies will spread a bit, so you may want to add 1 or 2 tablespoons (7 or 14 g) of almond flour.

Nutritional Information | Calories: 236 | Total Carbs: 8.9 g | Dietary Fiber: 5.2 g | Protein: 13.6 g | Fat: 20.2 g | Saturated Fat: 3.6 g

Banana Bread Mug Cakes

Banana-free banana bread? Yes, it does exist! These easy protein mug cakes are moist and delicious, and they take under 10 minutes to make.

Yield: 2 servings

Prep Time: 5 minutes

Cook Time: 2 minutes

Total Time: 7 minutes

NUT-FREE, VEGETARIAN

6 tablespoons (45 g) whey protein powder

2 tablespoons (24 g) granular sweetener

1 tablespoon (7 g) coconut flour

½ teaspoon baking powder

Pinch salt

½ cup (120 g) high-protein yogurt

1 large egg

2 tablespoons (28 ml) avocado oil

1 tablespoon (15 ml) water

1 to 2 teaspoons banana extract

½ teaspoon vanilla extract

1 tablespoon (15 g) sugar-free chocolate chips (optional)

1. In a small bowl, whisk the protein powder, sweetener, coconut flour, baking powder, and salt to blend.

2. In a medium bowl, whisk the yogurt, egg, oil, water, banana extract, and vanilla. Add the dry ingredients to the wet ingredients and whisk until no lumps remain. Divide the batter between 2 large (6-ounce, or 170 ml) ramekins or mugs. Sprinkle the tops with the chocolate chips (if using).

3. Microwave each cake individually on high power for 60 to 90 seconds until the top is just set. The cake will rise quite a bit during cooking, but will fall as it cools.

Tips

You aren't locked in to banana flavor here. Use any extract or flavoring to change up this easy recipe. If you don't need to be nut-free, add some chopped pecans or walnuts!

Protein powder options

- I recommend whey protein or a vegan protein for this recipe, as egg white might make it a little rubbery. Collagen protein won't give this recipe a full amino acid profile. And keep in mind that plain hemp protein has a very strong flavor, which may overpower the extracts.

- If you use vanilla protein powder, leave out the vanilla extract and cut the sweetener back to 1 tablespoon (12 g).

Nutritional Information | Calories: 278 | Total Carbs: 9.3 g | Dietary Fiber: 6 g | Protein: 24.2 g | Fat: 22.6 g | Saturated Fat: 5 g

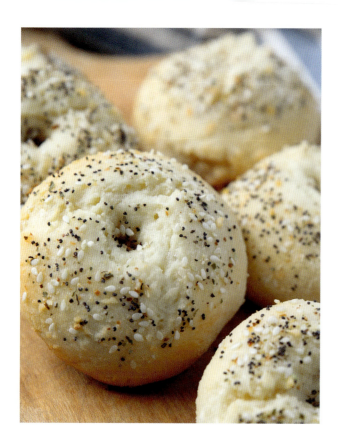
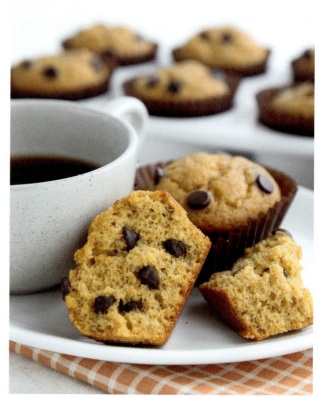
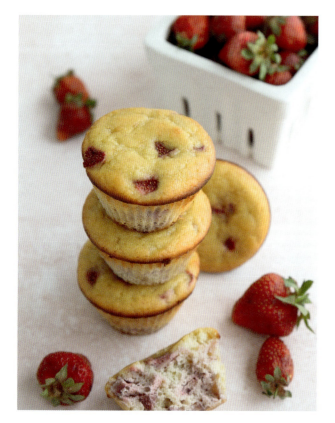
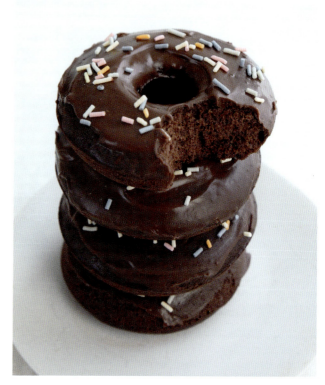

CHAPTER 5

BREADS AND MUFFINS

Want to know the secret to sticking with a healthy low-carb, high-protein diet? Muffins! As silly as that may sound, protein muffins have saved me from falling off the wagon on multiple occasions. They are easy to make, easy to freeze, and always delicious. I try to have some on hand at all times. And I love packing a few Pumpkin Spice Chocolate Chip Muffins (page 87) or Maple Walnut Muffins (page 91) with me when I travel.

Quick breads and donuts are also easy to bake in advance, which makes them perfect for meal prep. The Easy Protein Bagels (page 75) are great for sandwiches, and the Rustic Nut and Seed Bread (page 76) is delicious toasted up for breakfast. Try the Lemon Yogurt Loaf (page 78) with an afternoon coffee or enjoy it as dessert.

All the recipes in this chapter can help round out the protein content of other meals. Or you can enjoy them on their own to help increase your overall protein consumption.

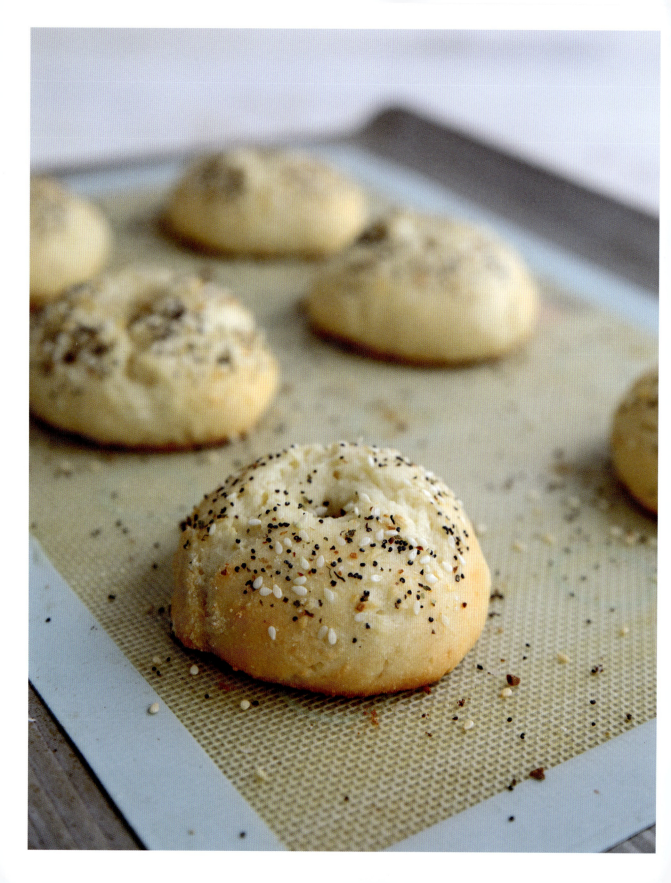

Easy Protein Bagels

Cottage cheese gives these low-carb bagels a wonderful texture and flavor. They're easy to make, have 13 grams of protein per serving, and are perfect for breakfast or lunch.

Yield: 6 bagels (1 bagel per serving)

Prep Time: 20 minutes

Cook Time: 22 minutes

Total Time: 42 minutes

VEGETARIAN

¾ cup (169 g) whole milk cottage cheese

2 large egg whites

1 cup (112 g) almond flour

⅓ cup (40 g) unflavored protein powder

2 tablespoons (14 g) coconut flour

2 teaspoons baking powder

¼ teaspoon salt

1½ teaspoons unsalted butter, melted

1 tablespoon (12 g) everything bagel seasoning

Protein powder options

Whey protein or egg white protein work best for this recipe.

1. Preheat the oven to 350°F (180°C or gas mark 4) and line a baking sheet with a silicone mat.

2. Place the cottage cheese in a blender and blend until smooth. Transfer to a large bowl and whisk in the egg whites until well combined. Add the almond flour, protein powder, coconut flour, baking powder, and salt. Work into a well-formed dough.

3. Wet or oil your hands and form the dough into 6 large balls. Place the dough balls on the prepared baking sheet and flatten them with your palm to about 1½ inches (3.5 cm) thick.

4. Dip the end of a wooden spoon into some water and press it into the center of each mound. Move the spoon in a small circle to make the hole a little bigger.

5. Brush the tops of the bagels with melted butter and sprinkle with everything bagel seasoning.

6. Bake for 18 to 22 minutes until puffed and just beginning to brown. Let cool completely. Store in an airtight container in the refrigerator for up to 1 week.

Tips

- Having wet or greased hands is a MUST when shaping these bagels. The dough is a bit sticky, but you will be able to roll it into balls as long as you take this precaution. If your dough is so sticky that you still struggle, add a bit more flour.

- If you only have part-skim cottage cheese, drain it in a fine-mesh sieve set over the sink or a bowl for 1 hour to reduce the excess moisture.

Nutritional Information | Calories: 195 | Total Carbs: 7.4 g | Dietary Fiber: 3.3 g | Protein: 13.3 g | Fat: 10.5 g | Saturated Fat: 1.7 g

Rustic Nut and Seed Bread

This low-carb bread is reminiscent of hearty loaves of rustic farmer's bread. It has wonderful flavor and holds together well when sliced. And it's fabulous as toast!

Yield: 14 slices (1 slice per serving)

Prep Time: 15 minutes

Cook Time: 45 minutes

Total Time: 1 hour

DAIRY-FREE OPTION, NUT-FREE OPTION, VEGETARIAN

- ⅓ cup (40 g) chopped walnuts
- ¼ cup (40 g) hemp seeds
- ¼ cup (36 g) shelled sunflower seeds
- 2 tablespoons (14 g) caraway seeds
- ¾ cup (83 g) pumpkin seed meal
- ½ cup (56 g) coconut flour
- ½ cup (60 g) unflavored whey protein powder
- 3 tablespoons (36 g) granular sweetener
- 1 tablespoon (14 g) baking powder
- ½ teaspoon salt
- 4 large egg whites
- 2 large eggs
- ¼ cup (60 ml) olive oil
- ¼ to ½ cup (60 to 120 ml) water

1. Preheat the oven to 325°F (170°C or gas mark 3) and lightly grease an 8 × 4-inch (20 × 10 cm) metal loaf pan. Line the bottom and long sides of the pan with parchment paper overhanging the edges for easy removal.

2. In a medium bowl, whisk the walnuts, hemp seeds, sunflower seeds, and caraway seeds to blend.

3. In a large bowl, whisk the pumpkin seed meal, coconut flour, protein powder, sweetener, baking powder, and salt to combine. Add about two-thirds of the nut and seed mixture and stir to combine.

4. Stir in the egg whites, eggs, oil, and ¼ cup (60 ml) of the water until well mixed. Add more water as needed to make a thick but scoopable batter. Spread the batter evenly in the prepared pan. Sprinkle with the remaining nut and seed mixture, pressing lightly to adhere.

5. Bake for 35 to 45 minutes until the top is golden brown and the center is just firm to the touch. Let cool completely in the pan, then lift out the bread using the overhanging parchment. Store the bread tightly wrapped on the counter for up to 4 days or in the refrigerator for up to 10 days.

Tips

- The caraway seeds give the bread a light rye flavor, which I love, but skip those, if you prefer. Switch out the walnuts for pecans or almonds or replace them with more seeds for a nut-free version.

Nutritional Information | Calories: 161 | Total Carbs: 5.8 g | Dietary Fiber: 2.8 g | Protein: 9 g | Fat: 11.2 g | Saturated Fat: 1.9 g

- When testing for doneness, always touch the top of the bread lightly. If it feels like it's mushy underneath, keep baking—but the moment it feels firm to the touch, get it out of the oven.

Protein powder options

This bread works well with whey or egg white protein powder. Vegan protein, for a dairy-free option, will work, but it will change the color and flavor of the bread. I don't recommend collagen for this recipe.

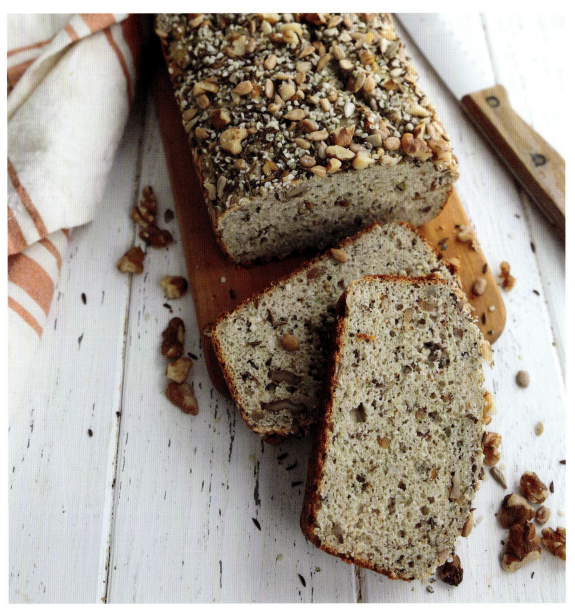

Lemon Yogurt Loaf

Love Starbucks Lemon Loaf but not the sugar? This tender high-protein quick bread has all the tangy lemon flavor you crave with only 5 grams of carbs per serving!

Yield: 12 slices (1 slice per serving)

Prep Time: 15 minutes

Cook Time: 45 minutes

Total Time: 1 hour

VEGETARIAN

FOR BREAD:

¾ cup (180 g) high-protein yogurt

3 large eggs

½ cup (96 g) granular sweetener

Grated zest of 1 lemon

1 teaspoon lemon extract

½ teaspoon vanilla extract

2 cups (224 g) almond flour

½ cup (60 g) whey protein powder

2 tablespoons (14 g) coconut flour, or another ⅓ cup (37 g) almond flour

2 teaspoons baking powder

¼ teaspoon salt

FOR GLAZE:

⅓ cup (43 g) powdered sweetener

1 to 2 tablespoons (15 to 28 ml) freshly squeezed lemon juice

1. Preheat the oven to 350°F (180°C or gas mark 4) and grease a 9 × 5-inch (23 × 13 cm) metal loaf pan. Line the pan with parchment paper with overhanging sides for easy removal and grease the parchment.

2. To make the bread: In a large bowl, whisk the yogurt, eggs, granular sweetener, lemon zest, lemon extract, and vanilla to blend.

3. Add the almond flour, protein powder, coconut flour, baking powder, and salt and stir until well combined. Pour the batter into the prepared pan and smooth the top.

4. Bake for 10 minutes, then reduce the oven temperature to 325°F (170°C or gas mark 3). Bake for 30 to 35 minutes more, or until the edges are golden brown and the top is just firm to the touch. Let cool completely in the pan, then lift out the bread using the parchment.

5. To make the glaze: In a medium bowl, whisk the powdered sweetener and 1 tablespoon (15 ml) of the lemon juice until smooth. Add more lemon juice, 1 teaspoon at a time, until the glaze is a drizzling consistency. Drizzle over the cooled bread and let set for 30 minutes before slicing. Store the bread tightly wrapped in the refrigerator for up to 1 week.

Tips

- Metal conducts heat much better than glass or ceramic bakeware, so it's the best choice for recipes like this. If you use glass or ceramic, reduce the oven temperature by 25°F (10°C). You may need to bake the bread longer to make sure it's cooked through.

Nutritional Information | Calories: 151 | Total Carbs: 5.4 g | Dietary Fiber: 2 g | Protein: 10.6 g | Fat: 10.8 g | Saturated Fat: 1.2 g

- Sweeteners that contain allulose will cause this bread to brown much faster, so keep an eye on it if you use them.

- You do not want to overbake recipes that contain protein powder, as they can become overly dry. Check on this bread frequently toward the end of the baking time. The minute the top feels firm to the touch, remove it from the oven.

Protein powder options

You can also use egg white protein powder for this recipe. Plant-based powder may work, but it will affect the color and flavor of the bread.

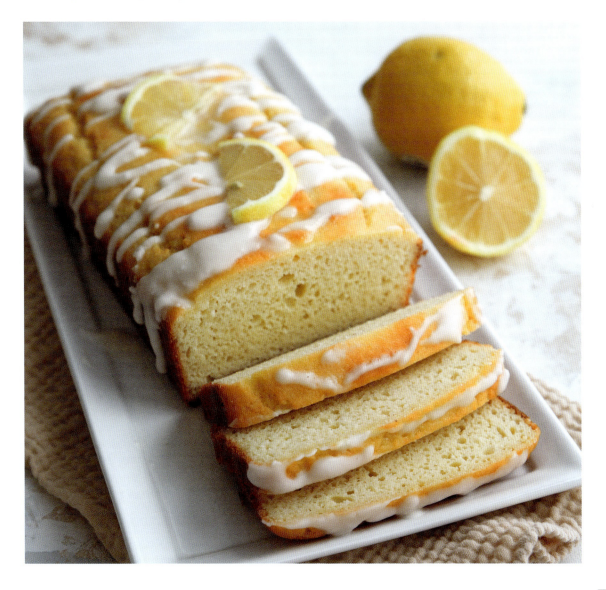

Double Chocolate Zucchini Bread

Zucchini adds wonderful moisture and tenderness to this rich chocolate bread. The chocolate chips don't hurt either!

Yield: 12 slices (1 slice per serving)

Prep Time: 15 minutes

Cook Time: 55 minutes

Total Time: 1 hour 10 minutes

DAIRY-FREE OPTION, VEGETARIAN

3 large eggs

½ cup (96 g) brown sugar substitute

⅓ cup (80 ml) avocado oil

1 teaspoon vanilla extract

2 cups (240 g) lightly packed shredded zucchini (not salted or drained)

1½ cups (168 g) almond flour

¾ cup (72 g) chocolate whey or (84 g) egg white protein powder (dairy-free option)

3 tablespoons (15 g) cocoa powder

1 teaspoon baking powder

½ teaspoon espresso powder (optional)

½ teaspoon salt

½ cup (120 g) sugar-free chocolate chips, divided

1. Preheat the oven to 325°F (170°C or gas mark 3) and grease a 9 × 5-inch (23 × 13 cm) metal loaf pan. Line the pan with parchment paper with overhanging sides for easy removal and grease the parchment.

2. In a large bowl, whisk the eggs, brown sugar substitute, oil, and vanilla until well combined. Whisk in the zucchini.

3. Add the almond flour, protein powder, cocoa powder, baking powder, espresso powder (if using), and salt and stir until well combined. Stir in about half of the chocolate chips. Pour the batter into the prepared pan and sprinkle with the remaining chocolate chips.

4. Bake for 45 to 55 minutes until the top is just firm to the touch. Let cool completely in the pan, then lift out the bread using the parchment. Store the bread tightly wrapped in the refrigerator for up to 1 week.

Tips

Espresso powder deepens the chocolate flavor in baked goods. It won't make this bread taste like coffee or mocha, but you are also free to skip it.

Protein powder options

- I tried this recipe with a few different kinds of protein powder. The first attempt was with beef isolate powder, and it rose beautifully and then sank as it cooled. It was more like brownies than bread, and

Nutritional Information | Calories: 200 | Total Carbs: 8.8 g | Dietary Fiber: 5.1 g | Protein: 11 g | Fat: 18.2 g | Saturated Fat: 4.6 g

while it was delicious, it wasn't quite what I was going for. I recommend sticking with whey or egg white, or possibly plant protein.

- If you don't have chocolate protein powder, add an extra tablespoon (5 g) of cocoa powder and another tablespoon (12 g) of sweetener.

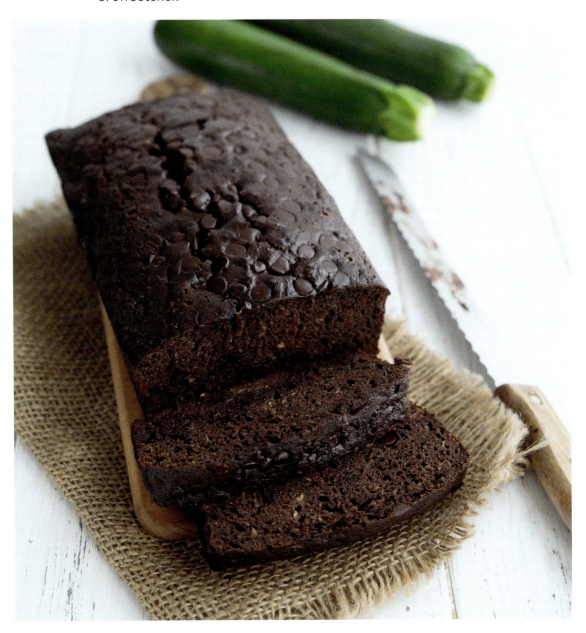

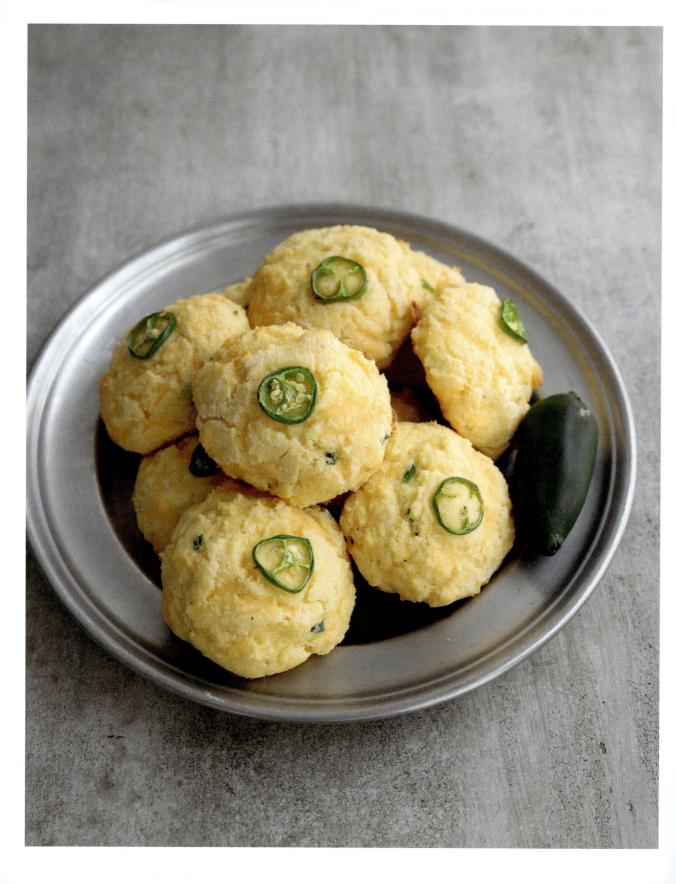

Cheddar Jalapeño Biscuits

Life is better with biscuits! These make a great side dish for lunch or dinner and a fabulous breakfast sandwich too.

Yield: 10 biscuits (1 biscuit per serving)

Prep Time: 15 minutes

Cook Time: 18 minutes

Total Time: 33 minutes

VEGETARIAN

1 cup (112 g) almond flour

½ cup (60 g) unflavored whey protein powder

¼ cup (28 g) coconut flour

2 teaspoons baking powder

½ teaspoon garlic powder

½ teaspoon salt

4 large eggs

½ cup (120 g) high-protein yogurt

3 ounces (85 g) cheddar cheese, shredded

1 medium-size jalapeño pepper, minced, plus 10 thin slices (optional)

1 tablespoon (14 g) salted butter, melted

Protein powder options

Unflavored whey protein is the best option for these biscuits. Other powders will make them too dry (egg white) or too gummy (collagen).

1. Preheat the oven to 375°F (190°C or gas mark 5) and line a large baking sheet with a silicone mat or parchment paper.

2. In a large bowl, whisk the almond flour, protein powder, coconut flour, baking powder, garlic powder, and salt to blend. Stir in the eggs and yogurt until the dough comes together, then stir in the cheese and minced jalapeño. Scoop the dough into 10 even mounds onto the prepared baking sheet. Use lightly wet hands to shape them into rounded, tall mounds, 1½ to 2 inches (3.5 to 5 cm) high.

3. Brush the mounds with melted butter and gently press 1 jalapeño slice into the top of each (if using).

4. Bake for 15 to 18 minutes until the tops are light golden and just firm to the touch. Let cool on the pan.

5. Store the biscuits in an airtight container in the refrigerator for up to 1 week.

Tips

Shaping the biscuits into taller mounds helps them keep their shape and spread less during baking. Have your hands just a little wet so the dough doesn't stick. You do not have to add the jalapeños if you don't like things spicy. Try cheddar and chives or cheddar and bacon. You can also make them as plain biscuits.

Nutritional Information | Calories: 174 | Total Carbs: 5.3 g | Dietary Fiber: 2.3 g | Protein: 12.9 g | Fat: 11.7 g | Saturated Fat: 4 g

Egg White Wraps

These homemade egg white wraps are perfect for high-protein lunches. They are flexible yet sturdy enough to hold your favorite fillings. Chicken salad, tuna salad, turkey and cheese, the possibilities are endless! These wraps also make great low-carb noodles—slice them into strips and serve with a hearty Bolognese sauce for a high-protein dinner!

Yield: 6 wraps (1 wrap per serving)

Prep Time: 5 minutes

Cook Time: 20 minutes

Total Time: 25 minutes

DAIRY-FREE OPTION, NUT-FREE, VEGETARIAN

1 cup (240 g) egg whites (carton or fresh)

¼ cup (30 g) unflavored protein powder

½ teaspoon xanthan gum

¼ teaspoon garlic powder (optional)

Pinch salt

Avocado oil, for cooking

Protein powder options

I tried this recipe with both whey and hemp protein powders. Both worked well, but the hemp wraps had a grayish color. Egg white protein powder should also work.

1. In a blender or food processor, combine the egg whites, protein powder, xanthan gum, garlic powder (if using), and salt. Blend on low speed to combine.

2. Heat a 7- to 8-inch (18 to 20 cm) nonstick skillet over low heat and brush it lightly with oil. Once hot, pour ¼ cup (60 ml) of the egg white mixture into the center of the pan and swirl the pan to cover most of the pan's bottom. Cook until the edges are dry and curling, 1 to 2 minutes. Wiggle a thin spatula underneath one edge to lift it. Use your fingers to peel the wrap gently from the pan and flip it over. Cook for another minute or so on the other side, then transfer to a wire rack to cool.

3. Repeat with the remaining batter, greasing the pan lightly between wraps.

4. Store the wraps in an airtight container in the refrigerator for up to 4 days. They will stay flexible and soft.

Tips

- There is no question that making these wraps takes a little practice. The first one always comes out a bit misshapen for me, but then I get the hang of it.

- Use a nonstick skillet and grease it very lightly. I just brush it with a little avocado oil.

- Use your hands. I find I can peel the wraps gently from the surface with my fingers more easily than flipping them with a spatula. I lift just the edge with the spatula, until I can grab it.

Nutritional Information | Calories: 36 | Total Carbs: 0.7 g | Dietary Fiber: 0 g | Protein: 8.3 g | Fat: 0.2 g | Saturated Fat: 0.2 g

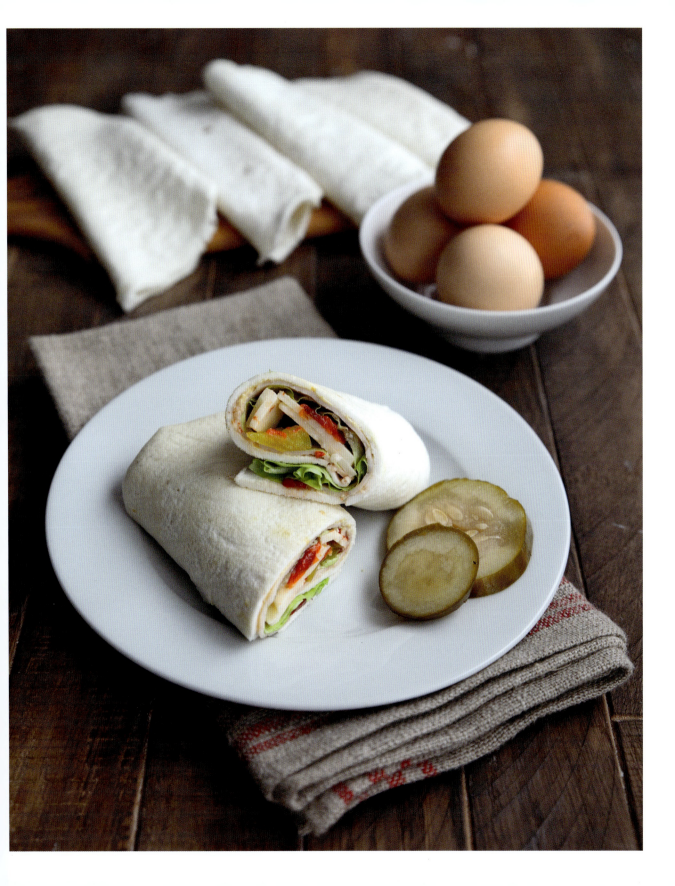

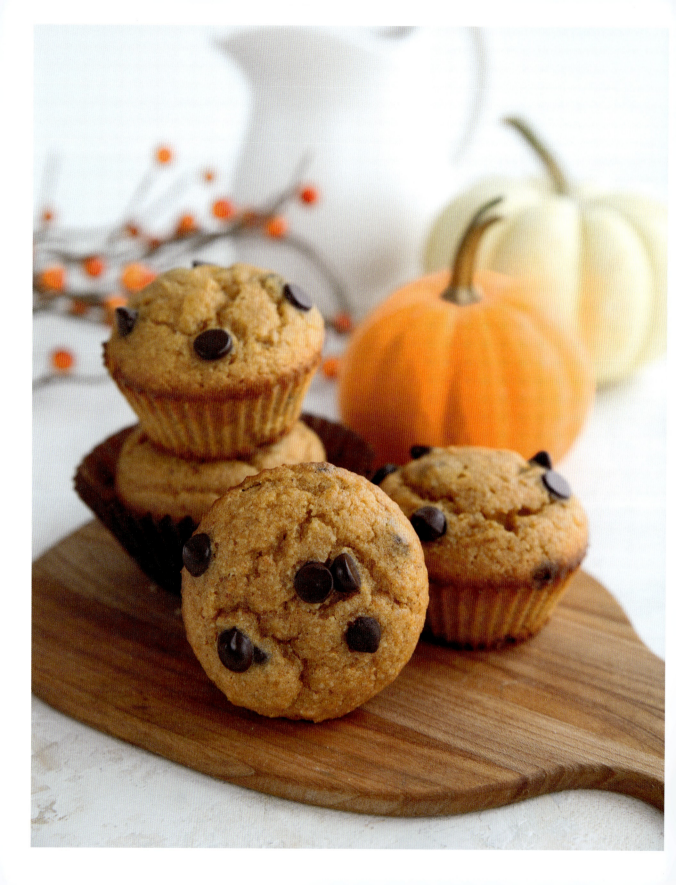

Pumpkin Spice Chocolate Chip Muffins

Who doesn't love a warm pumpkin muffin with hints of cinnamon and ginger? These tender muffins have all the flavor of your coffee shop favorite, with more protein and a fraction of the carbs.

Yield: 10 muffins (1 muffin per serving)

Prep Time: 15 minutes

Cook Time: 30 minutes

Total Time: 45 minutes

DAIRY-FREE OPTION, NUT-FREE, VEGETARIAN

⅔ cup (160 g) pumpkin purée

⅔ cup (128 g) brown sugar substitute

2 large eggs

¼ cup (60 ml) avocado oil

2 teaspoons vanilla extract

1½ cups (165 g) pumpkin seed meal (nut-free) or (168 g) almond flour

½ cup (60 g) whey protein powder

2 teaspoons pumpkin pie spice

1 teaspoon baking powder

½ teaspoon salt

⅓ cup (80 g) sugar-free chocolate chips (optional)

1. Preheat the oven to 325°F (175°C or gas mark 3) and line a standard muffin tin with 10 silicone or parchment paper liners.

2. In a large bowl, whisk the pumpkin, brown sugar substitute, eggs, oil, and vanilla to blend. Add the pumpkin seed meal, protein powder, pumpkin pie spice, baking powder, and salt and stir until well combined. Stir in the chocolate chips (if using).

3. Divide the batter evenly among the prepared muffin cups, filling each about three-quarters full.

4. Bake for 25 to 30 minutes until risen and just firm to the touch. Do not overbake. The muffins may still look a little wet in the center. Let cool completely in the pan. Store the muffins in an airtight container on the counter for up to 4 days or in the refrigerator for up to 1 week.

Tips

Although I prefer these muffins with a brown sugar substitute, they will work with any sweetener. Allulose may make them darken faster, so keep an eye on them in the oven.

Protein powder options

You can use egg white protein or plant-based protein for a dairy-free option, instead of whey protein. You can also use a flavored protein powder, such as vanilla, but choose one that doesn't contain sugar or reduce the sweetener to ⅓ cup (64 g), and skip the vanilla extract.

Nutritional Information | Calories: 189 | Total Carbs: 8 g | Dietary Fiber: 3.3 g | Protein: 10.8 g | Fat: 14.9 g | Saturated Fat: 2.7 g

Strawberry Vanilla Muffins

Start your day with these tender vanilla-scented muffins bursting with fresh berries. They're made with coconut flour, so they are completely nut-free too!

Yield: 10 muffins (1 muffin per serving)

Prep Time: 15 minutes

Cook Time: 30 minutes

Total Time: 45 minutes

NUT-FREE, VEGETARIAN

- ⅔ cup (160 g) high-protein yogurt
- 3 large eggs
- 1 large egg white
- ½ cup (96 g) granular sweetener
- 2 tablespoons (28 ml) avocado oil
- ⅔ cup (80 g) vanilla protein powder
- ½ cup (56 g) coconut flour
- ½ teaspoon baking soda
- ¼ teaspoon salt
- 1 cup (170 g) chopped fresh strawberries, divided

Protein powder options

This recipe works best with whey or egg white protein, but plant-based protein can work as well.

1. Preheat the oven to 325°F (170°C or gas mark 3) and line a standard muffin tin with 10 silicone or parchment paper liners.

2. In a large bowl, whisk the yogurt, eggs, egg white, sweetener, and oil until smooth. Add the protein powder, coconut flour, baking soda, and salt and stir until well combined.

3. Add about ¾ cup (128 g) of the strawberries and stir until well distributed. Divide the batter among the prepared muffin cups, filling each almost to the top. Top the muffins with the remaining strawberries.

4. Bake for 25 to 30 minutes, or until golden brown around the edges and the tops are just firm to the touch. Let cool for 15 minutes in the pan, then transfer the muffins to a wire rack to cool completely. Store the muffins in an airtight container in the refrigerator for up to 1 week.

Tips

- You can use vanilla-flavored protein powder and plain yogurt OR plain protein powder and vanilla yogurt. The vanilla quickly becomes overpowering if both ingredients are flavored.

- Try switching up the berries for a different flavor profile. Both fresh blueberries and raspberries are delicious.

Nutritional Information | Calories: 100 | Total Carbs: 5.7 g | Dietary Fiber: 2.3 g | Protein: 10.8 g | Fat: 5.2 g | Saturated Fat: 1.9 g

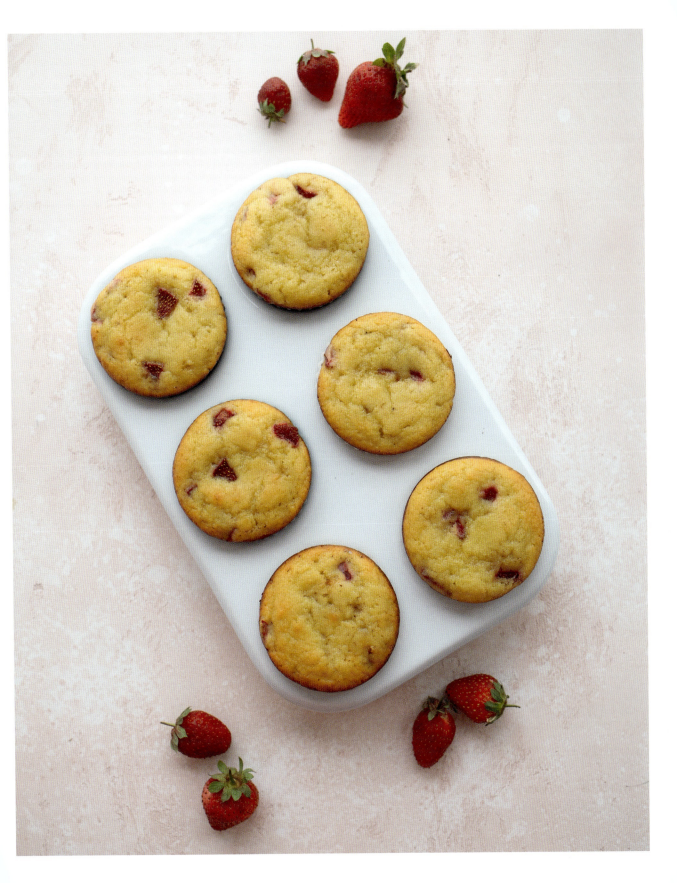

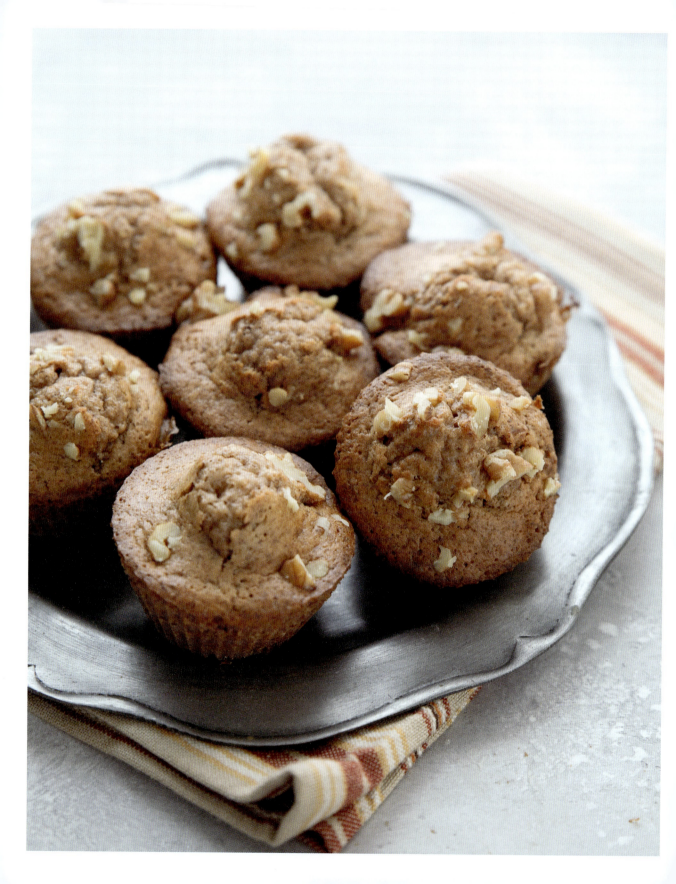

Maple Walnut Muffins

Maple and walnuts go so well together, and it's one of my favorite flavor combinations—but real maple syrup is not exactly low-carb friendly. Thank goodness for maple extract! My pantry is never without a bottle. And because walnuts and almonds contain tryptophan, this recipe offers the full complement of amino acids.

Yield: 12 muffins (1 muffin per serving)

Prep Time: 15 minutes

Cook Time: 25 minutes

Total Time: 40 minutes

FOR MUFFINS:

1 cup (260 g) almond butter

1 tablespoon (14 g) unsalted butter

½ cup (96 g) brown sugar substitute

1 teaspoon maple extract

3 large eggs

½ cup (56 g) collagen protein powder

2 teaspoons baking powder

¼ teaspoon salt

½ cup (60 g) chopped walnuts, divided

FOR DRIZZLE (OPTIONAL):

¼ cup (32 g) powdered sweetener

1 tablespoon (15 ml) heavy whipping cream

1 teaspoon maple extract

Water, as needed

Protein powder options
This recipe requires collagen or bone broth protein to work properly.

1. Preheat the oven to 350°F (180°C or gas mark 4) and line a standard muffin tin with 12 silicone or parchment paper liners.

2. To make the muffins: Place the almond butter and butter in a large microwave-safe bowl and microwave on full power until they are melted and can be stirred together, 30 to 60 seconds. Alternatively, melt them in a pan over low heat. Whisk in the brown sugar substitute and maple extract until well combined, then whisk in the eggs. Add the collagen powder, baking powder, and salt and stir until well combined. Stir in two-thirds of the walnuts. Divide the batter evenly among the prepared muffin cups and top with the remaining chopped nuts.

3. Bake for 18 to 25 minutes, or until the muffins have risen, are golden brown, and firm to the touch on top. Let cool completely in the pan.

4. To make the drizzle: In a small bowl, whisk the powdered sweetener, cream, and maple extract until smooth. Add water as needed to thin to a drizzling consistency. Drizzle over the cooled muffins. Store the muffins in an airtight container on the counter for up to 4 days or in the refrigerator for up to 1 week.

Tips
Not a fan of walnuts? Try pecans instead! And if you can't access maple extract, vanilla is delicious too.

Nutritional Information | Calories: 229 | Total Carbs: 5 g | Dietary Fiber: 2.5 g | Protein: 14.9 g | Fat: 16.4 g | Saturated Fat: 3 g

Chocolate-Glazed Donuts

Who can resist a tender chocolate donut with a delicious chocolate glaze? Not me!

Yield: 6 donuts (1 donut per serving)

Prep Time: 15 minutes

Cook Time: 20 minutes

Total Time: 35 minutes

NUT-FREE, VEGETARIAN

FOR DONUTS:

⅓ cup (80 g) high-protein yogurt

3 large egg whites

2 tablespoons (28 ml) melted unsalted butter

1 teaspoon vanilla extract

⅓ cup (32 g) chocolate protein powder

3 tablespoons (36 g) granular sweetener

3 tablespoons (21 g) coconut flour

2 tablespoons (10 g) cocoa powder

1 teaspoon baking powder

¼ teaspoon salt

FOR GLAZE:

¼ cup (60 ml) heavy whipping cream

1½ ounces (42 g) sugar-free chocolate chips

Sugar-free sprinkles, for garnish (optional)

Protein powder options

This recipe works best with whey, egg white, or plant-based protein.

1. Preheat the oven to 325°F (170°C or gas mark 3) and grease 6 wells of a standard donut pan.

2. To make the donuts: In a large bowl, whisk the yogurt, egg whites, melted butter, and vanilla to blend. Add the protein powder, sweetener, coconut flour, cocoa powder, baking powder, and salt and stir until well combined. Divide the batter evenly among the prepared wells of the pan.

3. Bake for 12 to 15 minutes until just barely firm to the touch. Let cool in the pan for 10 minutes, then flip the donuts onto a wire rack to cool completely.

4. To make the glaze: In a shallow microwave-safe bowl, heat the cream on high power until bubbling, about 15 seconds. Add the chocolate chips and let sit for 3 minutes to melt. Whisk until smooth and let the glaze cool and thicken for a few moments.

5. Dip the tops of the donuts into the glaze and place them back on the wire rack. Decorate with sprinkles (if using). Store the donuts in an airtight container on the counter for up to 4 days or in the refrigerator for up to 1 week.

Tips

- Don't have a donut pan? Make these in a standard muffin tin instead. Keep your eye on the muffins, as they may take slightly longer to bake.

- If you can't find sugar-free sprinkles, use chopped nuts or shaved chocolate.

Nutritional Information | Calories: 156 | Total Carbs: 7.1 g | Dietary Fiber: 3.8 g | Protein: 10 g | Fat: 10.3 g | Saturated Fat: 6.7 g

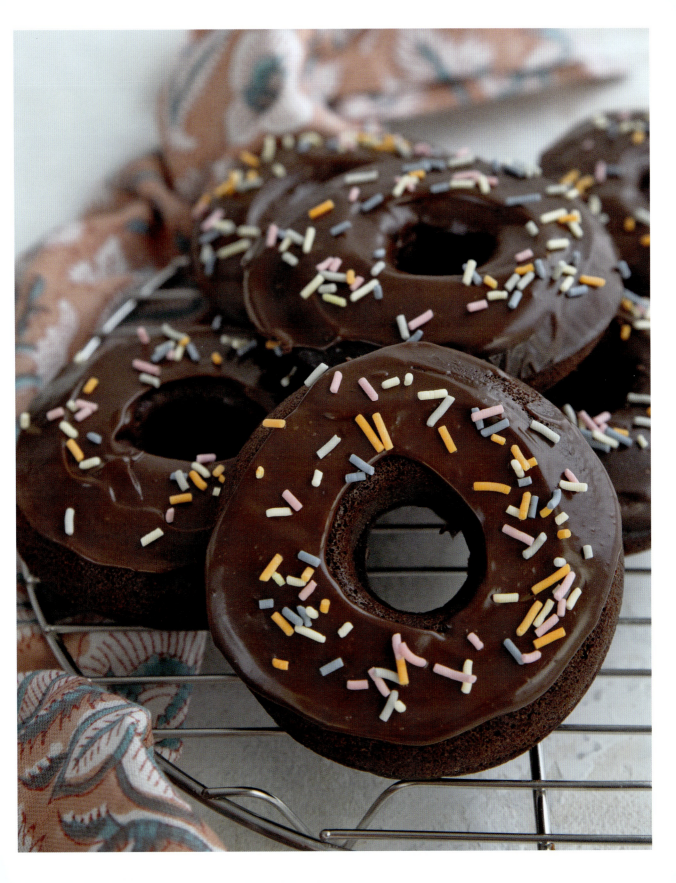

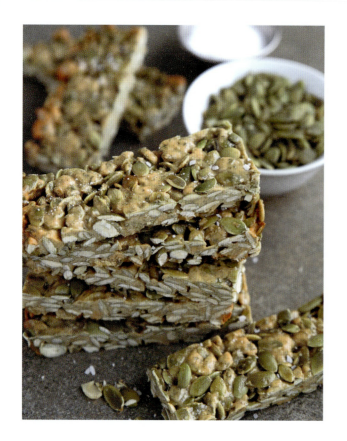

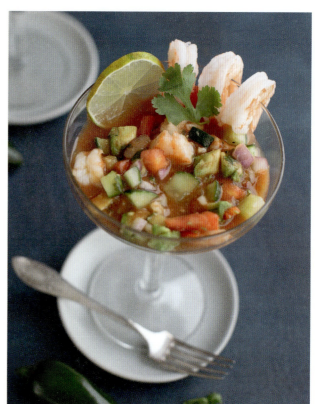

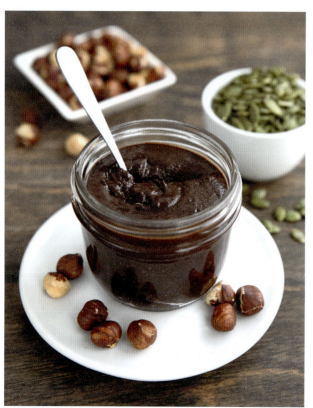

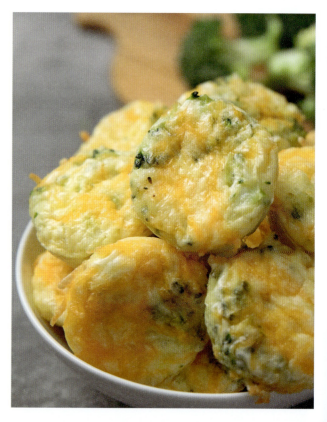

CHAPTER 6
APPETIZERS AND SNACKS

Used judiciously, snacks and appetizers can be a helpful tool on any healthy diet. While most of the nutrients and protein you consume should come from meals, snacks can bridge the gap and keep you on track when hunger strikes. They can also help top off a meal that's a little lighter in protein, allowing you to still meet your targets.

But overconsuming snacks can impede your health goals. Just because these recipes are low in carbs and high in protein doesn't mean that they are "free foods." Be mindful of how many you are eating and factor them into your daily consumption. If they are particularly tempting, try portioning them out in advance so you don't overdo it.

I love having easy grab-and-go snacks such as the Taco Bites (page 101) and the No-Bake Granola Bars (page 110) on hand. I often use them to top up my protein consumption at lunch or to quell the mid-afternoon munchies. My husband and I sometimes have a "date night" with appetizers and charcuterie, and the Easy 5 Seed Crackers (page 106) go so well with any cheese.

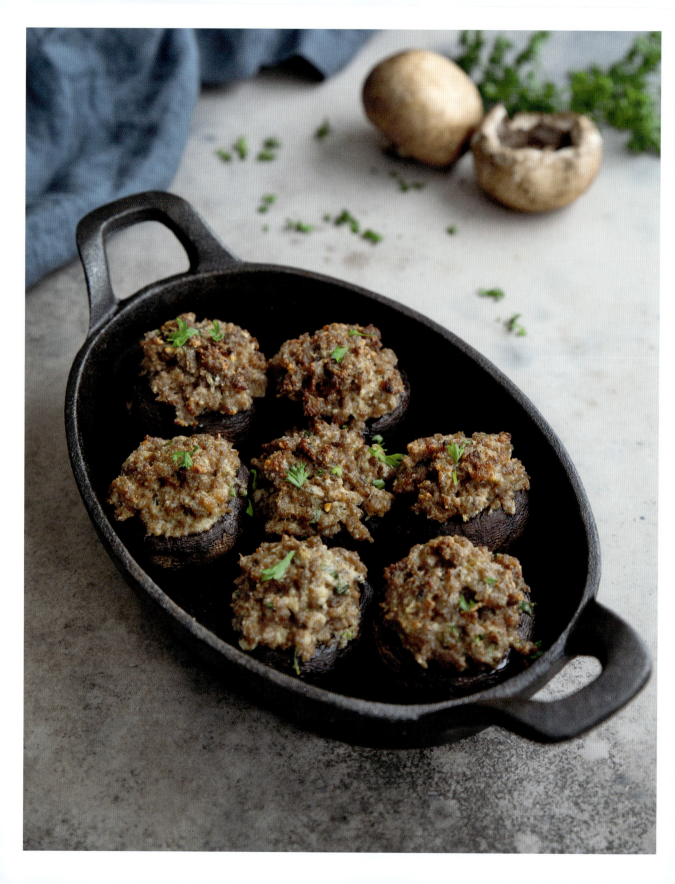

Sausage-Stuffed Mushrooms

Stuffed mushrooms are a classic appetizer for a crowd. If it's just you munching at home, make a half batch. Use hot or mild Italian sausage, as you like.

Yield: 10 servings

Prep Time: 20 minutes

Cook Time: 35 minutes

Total Time: 55 minutes

EGG-FREE, NUT-FREE

1 pound (455 g) cremini or button mushrooms

1 pound (455 g) bulk Italian sausage (pork, chicken, or turkey)

6 ounces (170 g) ricotta cheese

1 ounce (28 g) parmesan cheese, grated

2 garlic cloves, minced

1 tablespoon (4 g) chopped fresh parsley

1 teaspoon Italian seasoning

1. Preheat the oven to 400°F (200°C or gas mark 6).

2. With a damp cloth, wipe off any dirt from the outside of the mushrooms. Remove the stems. Use a small spoon to remove the gills from the inside of the mushrooms and place the mushrooms, hollow-side up, in a glass or ceramic baking dish.

3. In a large skillet over medium heat, brown the sausage until cooked through, about 10 minutes, breaking up any clumps with a wooden spoon. Use a slotted spoon to transfer the sausage to a bowl. Add the ricotta, parmesan, garlic, parsley, and Italian seasoning and stir well to combine. Spoon the filling into the hollows of the mushrooms, pressing it in to fill the whole cavity and mounding some on the top of each mushroom.

4. Bake for 20 to 25 minutes until the mushrooms are tender and the filling is nicely browned. Let cool for 10 minutes before serving.

Tips

- How many mushrooms you get depends on the size of the mushroom caps. I like slightly larger ones (2 inches, or 5 cm, across) because I can fill them more easily. Smaller mushrooms will also cook a little faster.

- Take the time to break up the sausage as it cooks. The smaller crumbles are easier to pack into the mushroom caps. If using chicken or turkey sausage, you may need to add a tablespoon (15 ml) of olive oil to the pan.

Nutritional Information | Calories: 207 | Total Carbs: 4.8 g | Dietary Fiber: 0.4 g | Protein: 12.8 g | Fat: 14.6 g | Saturated Fat: 6.3 g

Spanakopita Spinach Squares

These fun and tasty squares have all the flavor of your favorite Greek appetizer, with more protein and a fraction of the carbs.

Yield: 8 servings (2 squares per serving)

Prep Time: 15 minutes

Cook Time: 40 minutes

Total Time: 55 minutes

NUT-FREE, VEGETARIAN

12 ounces (340 g) frozen spinach, thawed

6 large eggs

1 cup (225 g) cottage cheese

¼ cup (40 g) finely diced onion

2 garlic cloves, minced

1½ teaspoons dried dill

½ teaspoon grated nutmeg

¼ teaspoon red pepper flakes

½ teaspoon salt

½ teaspoon ground black pepper

⅓ cup (40 g) coconut flour

1 teaspoon baking powder

¾ cup (113 g) crumbled feta cheese, divided

1. Preheat the oven to 350°F (180°C or gas mark 4) and grease an 8 × 8-inch (20 × 20 cm) baking pan.

2. Drain the spinach and squeeze out the excess moisture.

3. In a large bowl, whisk the eggs, cottage cheese, onion, garlic, dill, nutmeg, red pepper flakes, salt, and black pepper to combine. Whisk in the coconut flour and baking powder until well combined.

4. Add the spinach and two-thirds of the feta and mix until well distributed. Spread the batter in the prepared pan and sprinkle the top with the remaining feta.

5. Bake for 30 to 40 minutes until the edges are golden brown and the top is set. Let cool completely before cutting into 16 squares. Store any leftovers in an airtight container in the refrigerator for up to 1 week.

Tips

I used a ceramic baking dish for these squares. You can use metal, but they may bake faster and get more browned around the edges.

Nutritional Information | Calories: 143 | Total Carbs: 6.2 g | Dietary Fiber: 2.7 g | Protein: 12.2 g | Fat: 7.5 g | Saturated Fat: 4.4 g

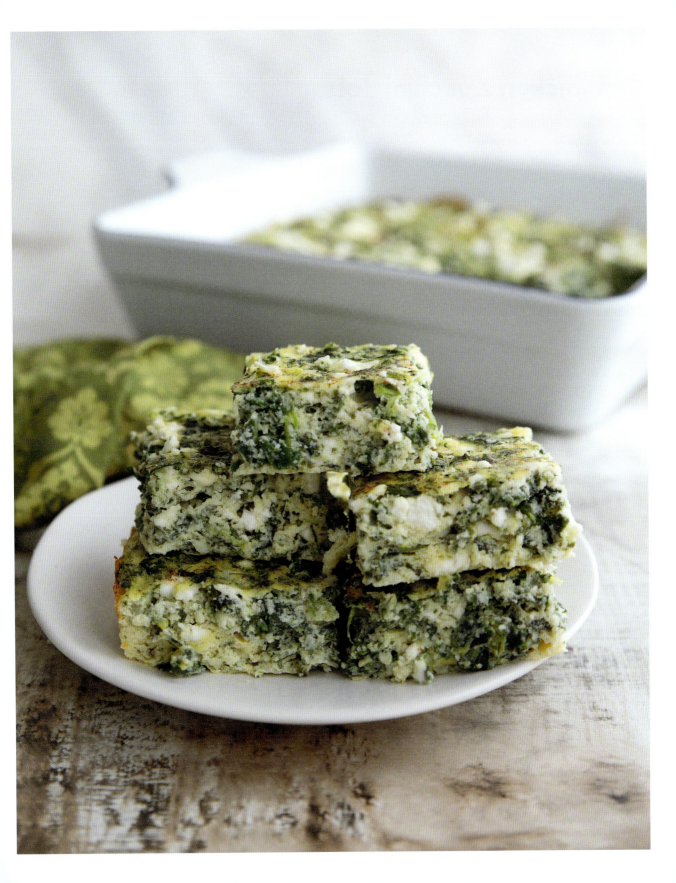

Chicken Zucchini Tots

These fun little chicken and zucchini "tots" are easy to make and can be served as an appetizer or a main dish. Dip them in sugar-free ketchup or ranch dressing.

Yield: 18 tots (3 tots per serving)

Prep Time: 1 hour 15 minutes (includes 1 hour to drain)

Cook Time: 10 minutes

Total Time: 1 hour 25 minutes

EGG-FREE, NUT-FREE

- 1½ cups (180 g) shredded zucchini
- ¾ teaspoon salt, divided
- 1 pound (455 g) ground chicken
- 4 garlic cloves, minced
- 2 ounces (55 g) cheddar cheese, shredded
- 2 tablespoons (14 g) coconut flour
- ½ teaspoon ground black pepper
- 1 tablespoon (14 g) unsalted butter, melted

1. Place the zucchini in a sieve set in the sink or over a large bowl and sprinkle with ¼ teaspoon of the salt. Toss to combine and let drain for 1 hour. Squeeze out as much moisture as possible.

2. In a large bowl, combine the zucchini, ground chicken, garlic, cheddar, and coconut flour. Add the remaining ½ teaspoon salt and the pepper. Mix well to combine. Use about 1½ tablespoons (25 ml) at a time to form the mixture into little tots or nuggets. You should be able to make 18 small tots.

3. Preheat an air fryer to 375°F (190°C).

4. Lightly grease the rack of an air fryer and add as many tots as will fit without crowding them. Brush the tops with melted butter.

5. Air fry for 8 to 10 minutes until golden brown. Alternatively, place the tots on a wire rack set on a baking sheet and bake at 375°F (190°C) for 15 to 20 minutes until golden brown.

Tips
Ground chicken can get very dry when overcooked. The zucchini helps, but make sure you keep an eye on them while cooking.

Nutritional Information | Calories: 188 | Total Carbs: 3.3 g | Dietary Fiber: 1.3 g | Protein: 26.3 g | Fat: 7.2 g | Saturated Fat: 4.2 g

Taco Bites

I made this recipe for a New Year's party a few years ago, and it was an instant hit with all my friends. Even the kids loved them! Serve with your favorite taco toppings, such as salsa, sour cream, and guacamole.

Yield: 32 bites (4 bites per serving)

Prep Time: 10 minutes

Cook Time: 30 minutes

Total Time: 40 minutes

NUT-FREE

1 pound (455 g) ground beef

3 tablespoons (27 g) taco seasoning

6 large eggs

1 cup (115 g) shredded cheddar cheese

1. In a large skillet over medium heat, sauté the ground beef until almost cooked through, about 8 minutes, breaking up any clumps with a wooden spoon. Stir in the taco seasoning and continue to sauté for 1 to 2 minutes more. Remove from the heat and let cool.

2. Preheat the oven to 350°F (180°C or gas mark 4) and generously grease a good nonstick mini muffin tin.

3. In a large bowl, whisk the eggs. Add the taco meat and the cheese and stir to combine. Fill the prepared muffin cups about three-quarters full with the meat mixture.

4. Bake for 15 to 20 minutes until puffed and firm to the touch. Let cool for 10 minutes. Run a thin flexible spatula around the edges of the muffins to release.

5. Store any leftovers in an airtight container in the refrigerator for up to 1 week.

Tips

- You can also use silicone or parchment mini muffin liners. If your pan is not very nonstick, this is the safest option. This recipe makes about 32 mini muffins, so you may need to work in batches if you only have one mini muffin tin. You could also cut the recipe down by one-third and make only 24 bites.

- If the taco seasoning you use is salt-free, add at least ¾ teaspoon salt to the beef.

Nutritional Information | Calories: 234 | Total Carbs: 1 g | Dietary Fiber: 0.2 g | Protein: 18.7 g | Fat: 14.5 g | Saturated Fat: 7.2 g

Broccoli Cheddar Bites

We like to keep these mini egg muffins in the fridge for quick protein snacks. You can also freeze them for several months. See bottom right of page 94 for photo.

Yield: 24 bites (6 bites per serving)

Prep Time: 15 minutes

Cook Time: 18 minutes

Total Time: 33 minutes

NUT-FREE, VEGETARIAN

2 cups (312 g) frozen broccoli florets, thawed

3 large eggs

2 large egg whites

½ cup (113 g) cottage cheese

1 teaspoon garlic powder

¾ teaspoon salt

½ teaspoon ground black pepper

2 ounces (55 g) cheddar cheese, shredded

1. Preheat the oven to 350°F (180°C or gas mark 4) and line a mini muffin tin with silicone or parchment paper liners.

2. Chop the broccoli florets into small pieces and divide evenly among the prepared muffin cups.

3. In a large bowl, whisk the eggs, egg whites, cottage cheese, garlic powder, salt, pepper, and cheese to combine. Spoon the egg mixture over the broccoli in the cups, filling them almost to the top.

4. Bake for 15 to 18 minutes until puffed and just firm to the touch. Let cool completely in the pan.

5. Store any leftovers in an airtight container in the refrigerator for up to 1 week.

Tips

- I recommend using muffin liners for these bites because they stick more than the Taco Bites (page 101) do.

Nutritional Information | Calories: 154 | Total Carbs: 4.4 g | Dietary Fiber: 1.2 g | Protein: 14.7 g | Fat: 8 g | Saturated Fat: 4.3 g

Mexican Shrimp Cocktail

This delightful dish is somewhere between pico de gallo, gazpacho, and shrimp cocktail. It has a bright, fresh flavor and looks extra appealing served in cocktail glasses. See top right of page 94 for photo.

Yield: 6 servings

Prep Time: 20 minutes

Total Time: 20 minutes

DAIRY-FREE, EGG-FREE, NUT-FREE

1 pound (455 g) cooked shrimp

½ medium-size cucumber, finely chopped

1 medium-size avocado, peeled, pitted, and finely chopped

1 medium-size tomato, finely chopped

¼ cup (40 g) chopped onion

¼ cup (4 g) chopped fresh cilantro leaves

½ medium-size jalapeño pepper, minced

2 garlic cloves, minced

¼ cup (60 ml) freshly squeezed lime juice

2 tablespoons (32 g) tomato paste

⅓ cup (80 ml) water

¾ teaspoon salt

½ teaspoon ground black pepper

1. Reserve 6 to 12 shrimp for garnish. Remove the tails and chop the remaining shrimp.

2. In a large bowl, stir together the chopped shrimp, cucumber, avocado, tomato, onion, cilantro, jalapeño, garlic, and lime juice.

3. In a medium bowl, whisk the tomato paste and water until well combined, add to the shrimp mixture, and toss to combine. Season with the salt and pepper. Divide the mixture among 6 cocktail glasses and garnish each with 1 or 2 of the reserved shrimp.

Tips

- You can make this recipe ahead and store it in an airtight container in the refrigerator for up to 3 days. Hold back on the salt and pepper if you are not serving it right away as it draws additional moisture out of the veggies and shrimp.

- Add more jalapeño if you like things on the spicy side.

Nutritional Information | Calories: 120 | Total Carbs: 6.5 g | Dietary Fiber: 2.3 g | Protein: 16.3 g | Fat: 3.4 g | Saturated Fat: 0.6 g

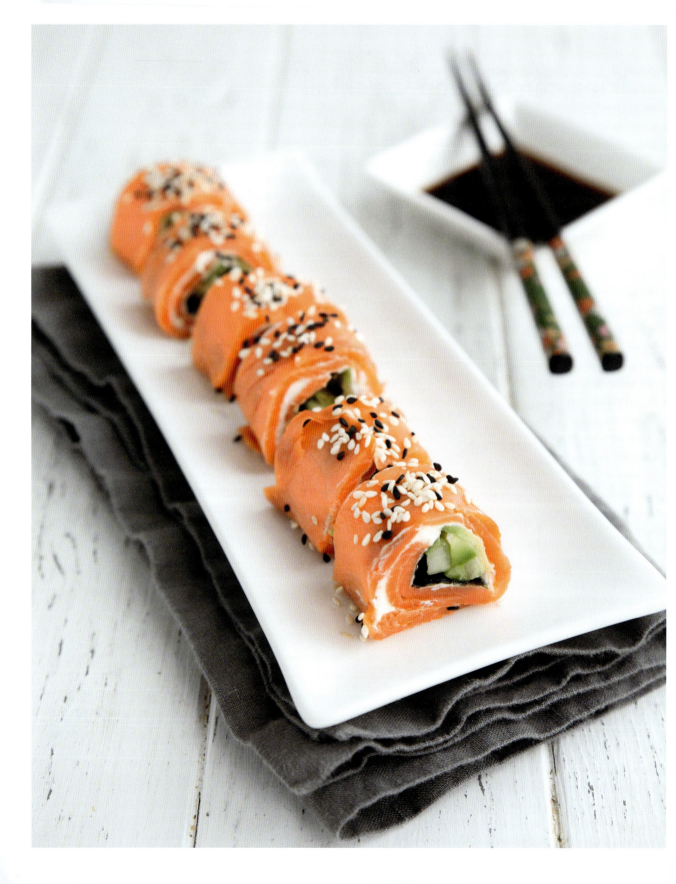

Smoked Salmon Sushi Rolls

These rice-free sushi rolls are easy to make and look elegant arranged on a white platter. It's one of my favorite high-protein snacks.

Yield: 2 servings (4 pieces each)

Prep Time: 35 minutes (includes 20 minutes to chill)

Total Time: 35 minutes

EGG-FREE, NUT-FREE

5 ounces (140 g) thinly sliced lox-style smoked salmon

2 ounces (55 g) cream cheese, softened

3 small seaweed sheets (from a package of seaweed snacks; optional)

¼ medium-size cucumber, cut into matchsticks

¼ medium-size avocado, peeled and thinly sliced

1 teaspoon toasted sesame seeds

Soy sauce, for serving (optional)

1. Lay a large piece of plastic wrap on a work surface. Arrange the salmon slices in an overlapping fashion to create a 6-inch (15 cm) square. Gently spread the cream cheese over the salmon. Lay the seaweed sheets (if using) along one edge of the square, then lay the cucumber and avocado on top of the seaweed.

2. Using the plastic wrap as a guide, roll the smoked salmon tightly around the fillings. Refrigerate the wrapped roll for 20 minutes to help firm it up.

3. Remove the plastic wrap and sprinkle the top of the roll with sesame seeds. Use a sharp knife to slice the roll into 8 even pieces. Serve with soy sauce (if using).

Tips

- This recipe scales easily to make more for a party or get-together. And you can make the rolls ahead and store, tightly wrapped, in the refrigerator for up to 3 days.

- Small seaweed sheets are the small rectangles that come in a package of seaweed snacks.

Nutritional Information | Calories: 221 | Total Carbs: 4.1 g | Dietary Fiber: 1.5 g | Protein: 16.5 g | Fat: 13.9 g | Saturated Fat: 6.7 g

Easy 5 Seed Crackers

I've always loved munching on crackers and cheese as an appetizer or easy snack. Having a high-protein option just makes it all the better. These crackers hold together nicely and store really well. And they are delightfully crispy.

Yield: 4 servings (about 8 crackers per serving)

Prep Time: 20 minutes

Cook Time: 45 minutes

Total Time: 1 hour 5 minutes

DAIRY-FREE, EGG-FREE, NUT-FREE, VEGETARIAN

½ cup (68 g) shelled pumpkin seeds

⅓ cup (48 g) shelled sunflower seeds

⅓ cup (37 g) flaxseed meal

¼ cup (36 g) sesame seeds

¼ cup (40 g) hemp seeds

¼ cup (31 g) unflavored hemp protein powder

1 teaspoon garlic powder

½ teaspoon kosher salt

¼ cup (60 ml) water, plus more as needed

Sea salt, for garnish

1. Preheat the oven to 325°F (170°C or gas mark 3).

2. In a large bowl, whisk the pumpkin seeds, sunflower seeds, flaxseed meal, sesame seeds, hemp seeds, protein powder, garlic powder, and kosher salt to combine. Add the water and use a rubber spatula to really work it into the seed mixture until a stiff dough forms. If the dough is too dry, add a little more water.

3. Lay a large piece of parchment paper on a work surface. Place the dough on the parchment and top with a second piece of parchment. Use a rolling pin to roll the dough to an even ¼ inch (6 mm) thickness. Remove the top piece of parchment, then use a sharp knife or a pizza wheel to score the dough into 2-inch (5 cm) squares. Transfer the parchment with the crackers to a large baking sheet. Sprinkle with a little sea salt.

4. Bake for 30 minutes. Remove from the oven and break off the edge pieces and any crackers that are firm and crisp. Continue baking the center pieces as needed until they crisp up, another 5 to 15 minutes.

5. Store the crackers in an airtight container at room temperature for up to 1 week.

Tips
- Rolling the dough as evenly as you can helps the crackers crisp up better. The edge pieces and outer crackers will always cook faster, so break them along the score lines when they are done and continue cooking the remaining crackers.

Nutritional Information | Calories: 181 | Total Carbs: 6.3 g | Dietary Fiber: 4.2 g | Protein: 9.9 g | Fat: 13.4 g | Saturated Fat: 1.8 g

- This recipe makes about 32 crackers (8 crackers per serving), but depending on how the dough is rolled and cut, that number can vary.

- If you live in a humid environment and your crackers soften, put them back into a warm (200°F or 93°C) oven for 10 minutes. They will crisp as they cool.

Protein powder options

I recommend hemp seed protein or egg white protein powder for this recipe. Whey protein will make the crackers softer and a bit more crumbly.

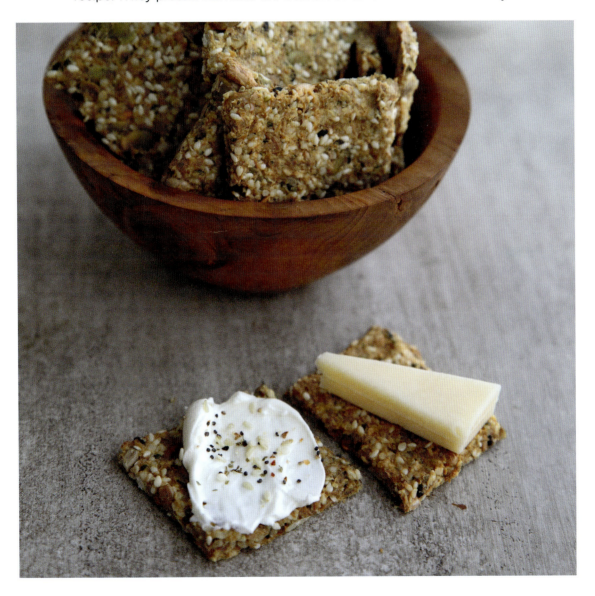

Brownie Protein Bars

Stop paying good money for outrageously priced protein bars that likely contain some questionable ingredients. It's so easy to make your own bars for quick snacks and post-workout fuel. These no-bake bars taste just like brownies.

Yield: 8 bars (1 bar per serving)

Prep Time: 1 hour 20 minutes (includes 1 hour to chill)

Total Time: 1 hour 20 minutes

DAIRY-FREE OPTION, EGG-FREE, NUT-FREE OPTION, VEGETARIAN

- ½ cup (130 g) creamy almond butter or other nut butter or seed butter (nut-free option)
- 1 teaspoon vanilla extract
- ¾ cup (72 g) chocolate protein powder
- ⅓ cup (43 g) powdered sweetener
- 3 tablespoons (15 g) Dutch-process cocoa powder
- 1 cup (110 g) pumpkin seed meal
- 2 to 4 tablespoons (28 to 60 ml) water
- 2 tablespoons (15 g) chopped walnuts (optional)

Protein powder options

For this recipe, you should be able to use almost any chocolate protein powder you like. The amount of water you need at the end will vary depending on the brand of protein, sweetener, and cocoa powder you use.

1. Line a 9 ×15-inch (23 × 38 cm) loaf pan with parchment or wax paper.

2. In a medium bowl, stir together the almond butter and vanilla until smooth. Add the protein powder, sweetener, and cocoa powder and mix until well combined.

3. Add the pumpkin seed meal and work it in with a rubber spatula. At this point, the dough may be a little crumbly. Stir in the water, 1 tablespoon (15 ml) at a time, until you have a thick dough that can be pressed together easily.

4. Press the dough into the prepared pan as evenly as possible. Use a flat-bottomed glass to smooth the top. Press the walnuts (if using) into the top. Refrigerate for 1 hour to firm up before cutting into 8 bars.

Tips

- If the almond butter has separated and has oil on the top, mix it in very well before measuring it. I like to dump the whole jar into my blender and blend it to recombine the oils. I find it will stay combined for several weeks in the fridge.

- I prefer to use a Dutch-process cocoa powder for recipes like this. It has a deeper chocolate flavor and combines better with the other ingredients.

Nutritional Information | Calories: 230 | Total Carbs: 8 g | Dietary Fiber: 3.2 g | Protein: 15.3 g | Fat: 16.1 g | Saturated Fat: 2.8 g

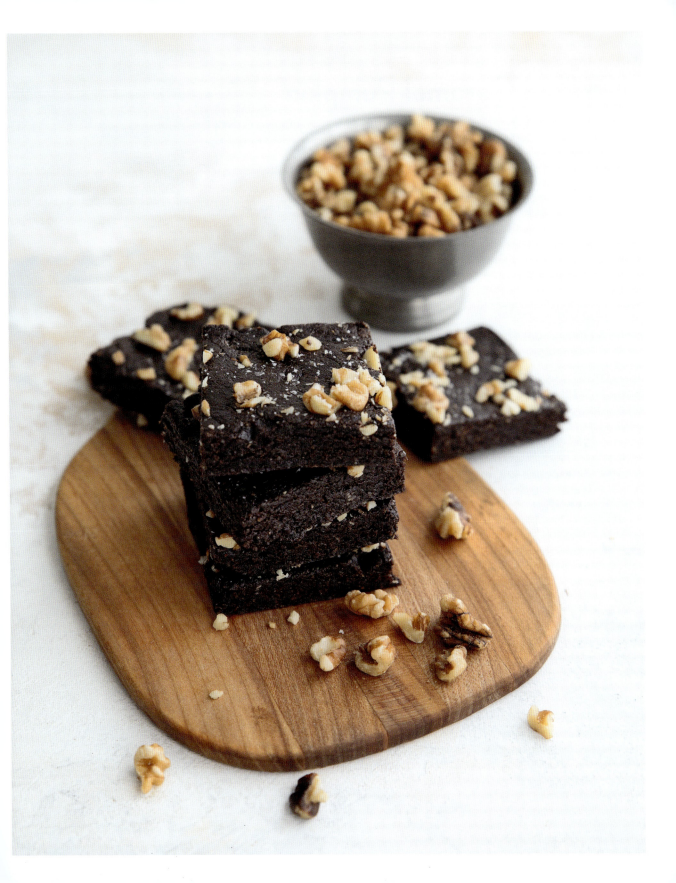

Salted Caramel Pumpkin Seed Bars

Sweet and salty goodness! These chewy snack bars are reminiscent of KIND bars, but without the added sugar. Feel free to drizzle a little sugar-free chocolate on top. See top left of page 94 for photo.

Yield: 10 bars (1 bar per serving)

Prep Time: 15 minutes

Cook Time: 20 minutes

Total Time: 35 minutes

DAIRY-FREE, NUT-FREE, VEGETARIAN

1¾ cups (238 g) shelled pumpkin seeds

½ cup (56 g) egg white protein powder

6 tablespoons (72 g) granular sweetener

¼ cup (28 g) pumpkin seed meal

½ teaspoon kosher salt

2 tablespoons (28 ml) avocado oil

2 tablespoons (28 ml) water, plus more as needed

1 teaspoon caramel extract

Sea salt, for garnish

Protein powder options

I tested these with both egg white and whey protein. They ended up firmer and chewier with the egg white, but the whey protein worked too. Plant-based protein would likely work, but collagen will make them too soft.

1. Preheat the oven to 300°F (150°C or gas mark 2) and line an 8 × 8-inch (20 × 20 cm) pan with parchment paper with overhanging sides for easy removal.

2. In a large bowl, whisk the pumpkin seeds, protein powder, sweetener, pumpkin seed meal, and kosher salt to combine.

3. Add the oil, water, and caramel extract and stir with a rubber spatula until the mixture clumps. You may need to really work the mixture together. If it's still too dry, add a little water, a few teaspoons at a time. Press the dough firmly into the prepared pan. Use a flat-bottomed glass to press it in evenly and smooth the top. Sprinkle with a little sea salt.

4. Bake for 18 to 20 minutes until golden around the edges and firm to the touch. Let cool completely in the pan, then lift out by the parchment and cut into 10 bars.

5. Store in an airtight container on the counter for up to 5 days or in the refrigerator for up to 10 days.

Tips

- If you can eat nuts, you can substitute almond flour, or any other nut meal, for the pumpkin seed meal. You can also use vanilla extract rather than caramel.

- Erythritol-based sweeteners will give you a crisp bar, whereas allulose and xylitol will make them softer.

Nutritional Information | Calories: 177 | Total Carbs: 3.1 g | Dietary Fiber: 1.5 g | Protein: 12.3 g | Fat: 14.3 g | Saturated Fat: 2.4 g

No-Bake Granola Bars

I've been making these easy no-bake bars for ages, and they are always a hit. The ground nuts and coconut give them a texture similar to no-bake oatmeal bars. Because the nuts and seeds contain tryptophan, these bars have a complete amino acid profile.

Yield: 16 bars (1 bar per serving)

Prep Time: 2 hours 15 minutes (includes 2 hours to chill)

Total Time: 2 hours 15 minutes

DAIRY-FREE OPTION, EGG-FREE, VEGETARIAN

1 cup (99 g) sliced almonds

¾ cup (45 g) unsweetened flaked coconut

½ cup (60 g) walnuts or (55 g) pecans

½ cup (68 g) shelled pumpkin seeds

⅔ cup (80 g) unflavored whey protein powder

⅓ cup (43 g) powdered sweetener

½ teaspoon salt

1 cup (260 g) creamy natural peanut butter or other nut butter

3 tablespoons (60 g) low-carb honey alternative

½ teaspoon vanilla extract

Water, as needed

Protein powder options

Use any protein powder here. Collagen or bone broth protein may make the bars a little softer and stickier.

1. Line a 9 × 9-inch (23 × 23 cm) metal baking pan with parchment or wax paper.

2. In a food processor, combine the almonds, coconut, walnuts, and pumpkin seeds. Pulse until they resemble oat flakes with a few larger pieces. Transfer to a bowl and add the protein powder, sweetener, and salt. Stir until well combined.

3. Add the peanut butter, honey alternative, and vanilla. Stir until the mixture begins to hold together. Add water, 1 tablespoon (15 ml) at a time, if necessary, to help the dough cling together. It should feel like thick cookie dough.

4. Press the mixture firmly and evenly into the prepared baking pan. Chill for 2 hours until firm, then cut into 16 bars or squares with a sharp knife.

5. Store in an airtight container on the counter for up to 5 days or in the refrigerator for up to 10 days.

Tips

There are a few brands of low-carb and keto-friendly "honey" alternatives, usually made with allulose. I like the brand All-u-Lose, but if you don't want to use that, simply add another 2 tablespoons (16 g) of powdered sweetener and some additional water to help the mixture hold together.

Nutritional Information | Calories: 262 | Total Carbs: 8.1 g | Dietary Fiber: 3.1 g | Protein: 12.8 g | Fat: 18.1 g | Saturated Fat: 3.2 g

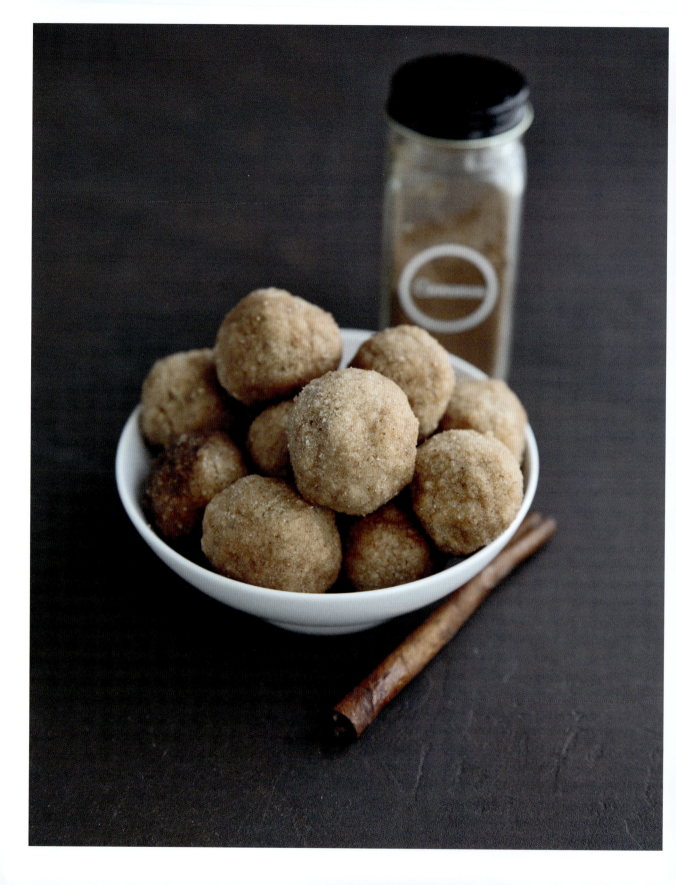

Snickerdoodle Protein Bites

Quick and easy protein balls that taste like snickerdoodle cookies?
Now that's my kind of protein snack!

Yield: 16 bites (2 bites per serving)

Prep Time: 30 minutes (includes 20 minutes to chill)

Total Time: 30 minutes

EGG-FREE, VEGETARIAN

⅔ cup (173 g) almond butter

¾ cup (90 g) unflavored whey protein powder

⅓ cup (43 g) powdered sweetener

¼ cup (28 g) almond flour

1½ teaspoons ground cinnamon, divided

1 teaspoon vanilla extract

¼ teaspoon cream of tartar

⅛ teaspoon salt

2 tablespoons (24 g) granular sweetener

1. Line a large plate with wax paper.

2. In a large bowl, stir the almond butter well to combine the oil and make it smooth.

3. Add the protein powder, powdered sweetener, almond flour, 1 teaspoon of the cinnamon, the vanilla, cream of tartar, and salt. Mix until a cohesive dough forms and you can roll it into firm balls. Divide the mixture into 16 portions and roll each into a ball, then place on the prepared plate. Refrigerate for 20 minutes to firm up.

4. In a small bowl, whisk the granular sweetener and remaining ½ teaspoon cinnamon. Roll the chilled balls in the cinnamon coating. Store in an airtight container in the refrigerator for up to 1 week.

Tips

- Depending on your almond butter and protein powder, the consistency of the dough may differ. However, it's easy to adjust: If your dough is too stiff and won't hold together, add a bit more oil. If the dough is too goopy and you can't roll it into balls, work in a bit more flour.

- Cream of tartar helps give these protein bites a classic snickerdoodle flavor. It is commonly found in the baking aisle among the spices. Skip it, if you prefer.

Nutritional Information | Calories: 187 | Total Carbs: 5.9 g | Dietary Fiber: 2.8 g | Protein: 13.8 g | Fat: 13.1 g | Saturated Fat: 1.9 g

Carrot Cake Protein Bites

Energy bites (a.k.a. protein balls) are a quick and easy way to get a little extra protein into your day. I like to have some in the refrigerator at all times for quick snacks or to help me round out a meal that's a little short on protein. This carrot cake version is entirely plant based.

Yield: 20 bites (2 bites per serving)

Prep Time: 50 minutes (includes 30 minutes to chill)

Total Time: 50 minutes

DAIRY-FREE, EGG-FREE, VEGETARIAN

¾ cup (75 g) pecans or walnuts or a mix

½ cup (30 g) unsweetened flaked coconut

3 tablespoons (45 ml) avocado oil

¾ cup (93 g) unflavored hemp protein powder

⅓ cup (43 g) powdered sweetener

1½ teaspoons ground cinnamon

½ teaspoon ground ginger

¼ teaspoon grated nutmeg

¼ teaspoon salt

1 cup (110 g) finely shredded carrots

⅓ cup (87 g) almond butter or other nut butter

Water, as needed

¼ cup (20 g) shredded coconut

1. Line a plate with wax paper.

2. In a food processor, combine the pecans, coconut, and oil and blend until the mixture starts to become a butter.

3. Add the protein powder, sweetener, cinnamon, ginger, nutmeg, and salt and pulse to combine. Use a rubber spatula to scrape down the sides of the processor.

4. Add the carrots and almond butter and pulse again until the mixture begins to clump together. Add water, 1 tablespoon (15 ml) at a time, until the mixture forms a stiff dough. Divide the dough into 20 portions and roll each into a ball.

5. Spread the shredded coconut on a shallow dish and roll the balls in the coconut. Place them on the prepared plate and refrigerate until firm, about 30 minutes. They can then be stored in an airtight container in the refrigerator for up to 1 week.

Tips

The mixture should be quite stiff, but you should be able to squeeze it in the palm of your hand and have it hold together. Don't add so much water that it becomes goopy!

Protein powder options

I tested these using a hemp protein blend, which gave them a bit of an earthy flavor. The recipe should also work using egg white, whey protein, or collagen.

Nutritional Information | Calories: 211 | Total Carbs: 6.4 g | Dietary Fiber: 3.5 g | Protein: 9.2 g | Fat: 19.2 g | Saturated Fat: 5.3 g

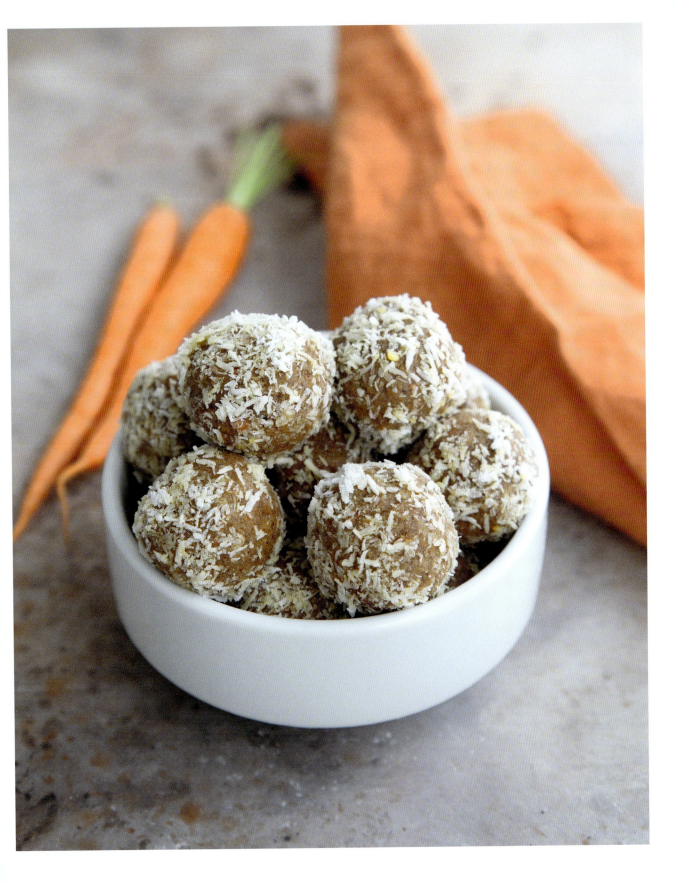

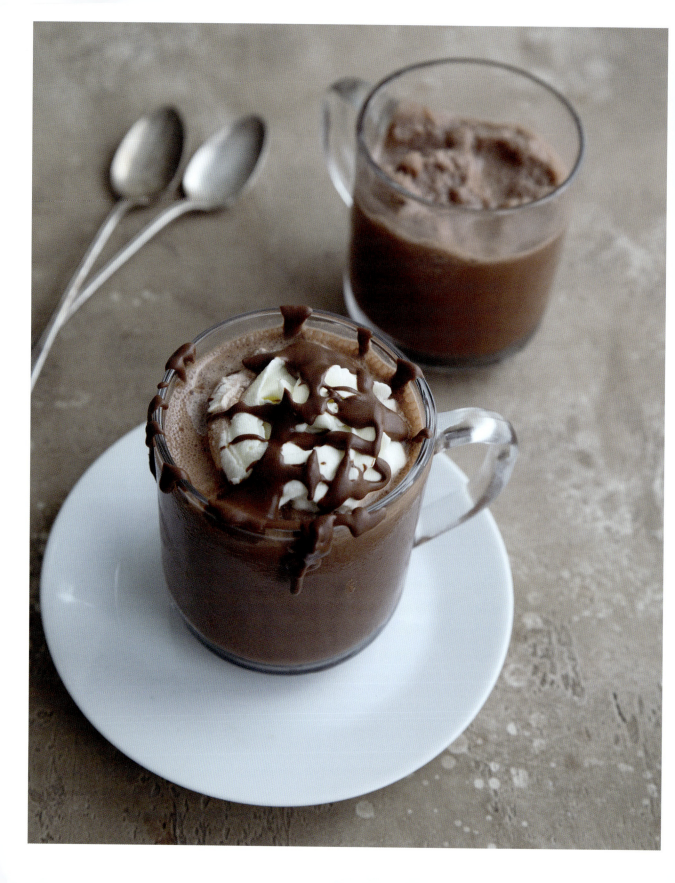

Frozen Hot Chocolate

It may sound like an oxymoron, but frozen hot chocolate is a real thing. It's usually made with premade hot chocolate mix, which of course contains plenty of sugar. My version is just as tasty and much better for you!

Yield: 2 servings

Prep Time: 10 minutes

Total Time: 10 minutes

EGG-FREE, NUT-FREE OPTION, VEGETARIAN

1 cup (217 g) crushed ice

¾ cup (175 ml) unsweetened almond or hemp milk (nut-free option)

⅓ cup (32 g) chocolate protein powder

2½ tablespoons (20 g) powdered sweetener, divided, plus more as needed

1 tablespoon (5 g) cocoa powder

½ teaspoon vanilla extract

¼ cup (60 ml) heavy whipping cream

1. In a blender, combine the ice, almond milk, protein powder, 2 tablespoons (16 g) of the sweetener, cocoa powder, and vanilla. Blend until smooth and creamy.

2. In a small bowl and using a handheld mixer, beat the cream with the remaining ½ tablespoon sweetener on medium-high speed until it holds stiff peaks.

3. Taste the chocolate mixture and add more sweetener as desired. Divide between 2 mugs and top with the whipped cream.

Tips
Crushed ice breaks up more easily in a blender, particularly if you don't have a high-speed version. Make sure to scrape down the sides of the blender jar a few times to mix everything well.

Protein powder options
This recipe should work with any kind of protein powder. If you only have plain powder, add another teaspoon or two of cocoa powder, then sweeten to taste at the end.

Nutritional Information | Calories: 197 | Total Carbs: 3.9 g | Dietary Fiber: 1 g | Protein: 17.6 g | Fat: 13.1 g | Saturated Fat: 7.7 g

Almond Joy Smoothies

These rich, dairy-free smoothies are an easy way to get a hit of protein. Fuel up after a workout or use them as a quick breakfast option.

Yield: 2 smoothies

Prep Time: 5 minutes

Total Time: 5 minutes

DAIRY-FREE, EGG-FREE, VEGETARIAN

¼ cup (60 ml) canned coconut milk

2 tablespoons (32 g) almond butter

½ cup (109 g) crushed ice

6 tablespoons (36 g) chocolate protein powder

1 tablespoon (5 g) cocoa powder

1 cup (235 ml) unsweetened almond milk

½ to 1 teaspoon coconut extract, plus more as needed

1. In a blender, combine all of the ingredients and blend until smooth. Taste and adjust the sweetness (see Tips) and coconut flavor as desired. Divide between 2 glasses and serve.

Tips

- Leave out any additional sweetener until you taste the smoothie, because many chocolate protein powders are very sweet.

- Coconut cream is the thick, white portion from the top of a can of coconut milk. You can actually purchase coconut cream, which has less liquid and water than coconut milk.

Protein powder options

Use any kind of protein you like best here (including whey, if you don't need to be dairy-free). If you only have unflavored protein, add 1½ teaspoons more cocoa powder and 1½ teaspoons of sweetener.

Nutritional Information | Calories: 256 | Total Carbs: 6.7 g | Dietary Fiber: 2.5 g | Protein: 23.2 g | Fat: 17.4 g | Saturated Fat: 7.4 g

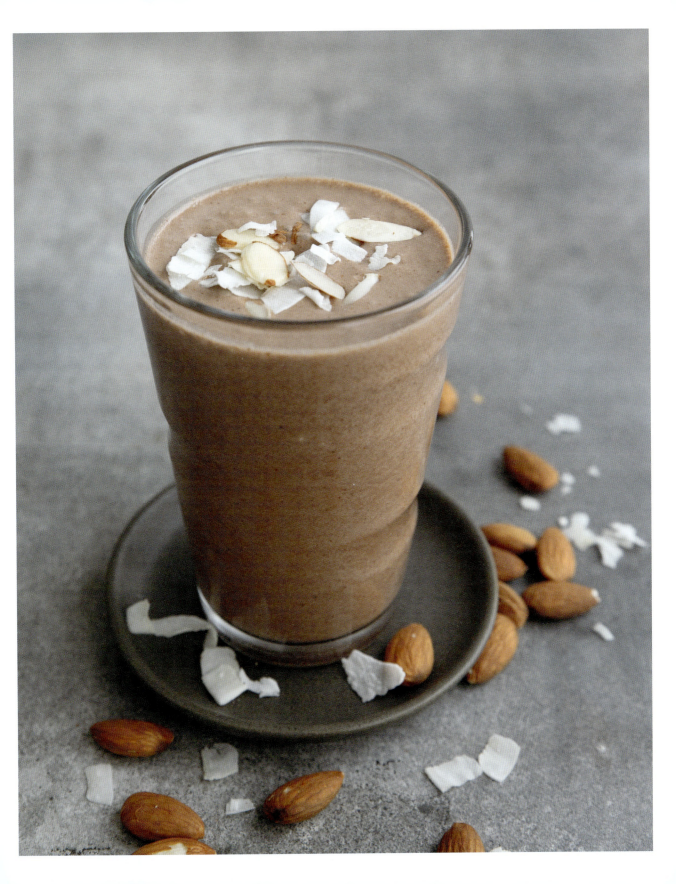

Pumpkin Spice Latte

I used to love sipping a PSL from Starbucks on a brisk fall day. Now I shudder to think at the astonishing amount of sugar I was consuming. I've been making my own sugar-free version for years, and I now add a hit of protein as well. Why not make my favorite fall beverage work a little harder for me?

Yield: 1 serving

Prep Time: 5 minutes

Cook Time: 5 minutes

Total Time: 10 minutes

EGG-FREE, NUT-FREE OPTION, VEGETARIAN

- 1 cup (235 ml) almond or hemp milk (nut-free option)
- 1 tablespoon (15 g) pumpkin purée
- 1 tablespoon (15 ml) heavy whipping cream
- ½ teaspoon pumpkin pie spice
- ½ teaspoon vanilla extract
- 2 teaspoons sweetener of choice, plus more as needed
- ¼ cup (30 g) unflavored whey protein powder
- ¼ cup (60 ml) brewed espresso or strong coffee
- Ground cinnamon, for garnish (optional)

1. In a small saucepan over medium heat, combine the almond milk, pumpkin purée, cream, pumpkin pie spice, vanilla, and sweetener. Bring to a simmer, whisking frequently. Remove from the heat and briskly whisk in the protein powder to combine and to froth the mixture. If you have a handheld frother, use that instead of a whisk. Taste and adjust the sweetener as desired.

2. Pour the coffee into a mug and add the frothed pumpkin cream. Sprinkle the top with cinnamon (if using).

Tips

- I use unsweetened almond milk to keep the carbs in check, but any low-carb milk will do. Hemp milk is a great option for a nut-free version.

- You can use almost any sweetener for this latte as long as it dissolves well. If you use a concentrated sweetener like stevia or monk fruit extract, add just the tiniest amount to start and adjust to taste.

Protein powder options

I prefer whey, egg white, or collagen protein for this recipe, as I find plant-based protein gives it an odd flavor. I also don't recommend flavored varieties, like vanilla, because they overpower the pumpkin spice.

Nutritional Information | Calories: 210 | Total Carbs: 4.3 g | Dietary Fiber: 0.6 g | Protein: 26.5 g | Fat: 10.9 g | Saturated Fat: 4.5 g

Chocolate Hazelnut Spread

This high-protein spread is delicious on low-carb bread, ice cream, or my Pumpkin Spice Chocolate Chip Muffins (page 87). If you're like me, you may just want to eat it with a spoon! See bottom left of page 94 for photo.

Yield: 6 servings
(2 tablespoons, or 32 g, per serving)

Prep Time: 10 minutes

Total Time: 10 minutes

DAIRY-FREE OPTION, EGG-FREE, VEGETARIAN

- ½ cup (68 g) shelled pumpkin seeds
- ⅓ cup (45 g) roasted unsalted hazelnuts
- 3 tablespoons (45 ml) hazelnut or avocado oil, divided, plus more as needed
- ⅓ cup (32 g) chocolate protein powder
- 3 tablespoons (24 g) powdered sweetener, plus more as needed
- 2 tablespoons (10 g) cocoa powder
- 1 teaspoon hazelnut extract
- ¼ teaspoon salt

Protein powder options

All varieties of protein powder work in this recipe. If you don't have a chocolate variety, use plain and add 1 additional tablespoon (5 g) cocoa powder and more sweetener to taste.

1. In a food processor or high-powered blender, combine the pumpkin seeds and hazelnuts. Process on high speed until they start to become nut butter, stopping to scrape down the sides of the bowl as needed. Add 1 tablespoon (15 ml) of the oil and continue to blend until smooth.

2. Add the protein powder, sweetener, cocoa powder, hazelnut extract, and salt. Blend until combined. The mixture may become very thick at this point. Add the remaining 2 tablespoons (28 ml) oil and blend until smooth and spreadable. Add more oil as needed and adjust the sweetness to taste.

Tips

- Using hazelnut oil and hazelnut extract intensifies the flavor; you can also use avocado oil, which is neutral in flavor, and vanilla extract.

- **How to roast hazelnuts:** I buy pre-roasted nuts if I can, but it's easy to roast them at home. Spread the nuts on a baking sheet and bake at 350°F (180°C or gas mark 4) for 10 minutes until lightly toasted. Once they are cool enough to touch, rub them between your fingers to take off most of the husks. Some of it will not come off and that's normal.

Nutritional Information | Calories: 164 | Total Carbs: 3.9 g | Dietary Fiber: 1.9 g | Protein: 9.8 g | Fat: 16.7 g | Saturated Fat: 2.6 g

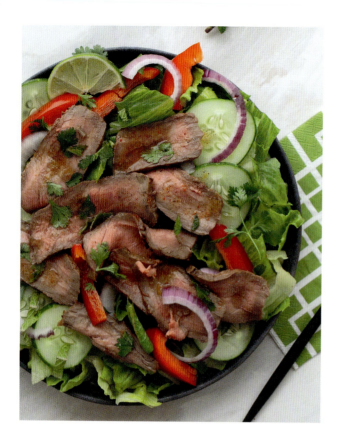

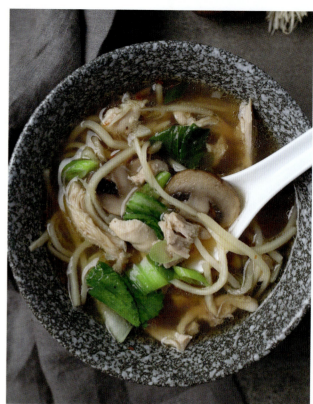

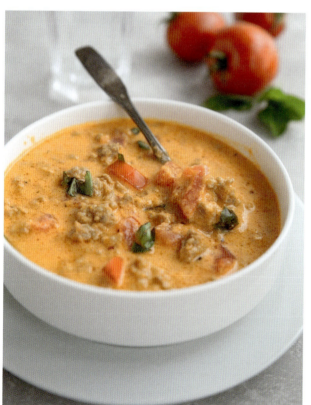

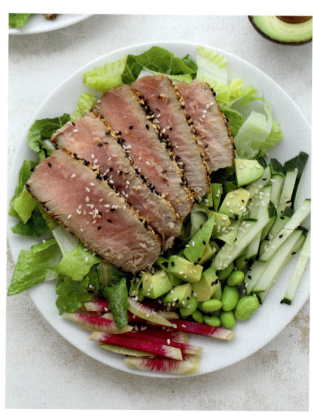

CHAPTER 7

SOUPS AND SALADS

I rely heavily on soups and salads for high-protein meals, and I encourage you to do the same. They are easy to pull together and full of high-quality nutrition. And they are often full meals unto themselves, replete with protein, good fats, and plenty of low-carb vegetables.

My husband and I make large entree-sized salads at least three times a week for easy lunches or dinners. To streamline the process, we purchase several heads of lettuce and wash and chop them in advance. I don't recommend bagged chopped lettuce, as it tends to get slimy rather quickly. When we prep the lettuce in advance, we can assemble recipes like the Turkey Club Salad (page 137) or the Thai Beef Salad (page 142) much more quickly.

Soups are a low-carb dieter's best friend. They are flavorful, comforting, and easy to prep ahead. They also make great meals any time of day—I often eat soup for breakfast on a chilly morning. I like to make big batches of Chicken Chile Verde (page 129) or Italian Beef and Vegetable Soup (page 126) and sock some away in the freezer for those "I don't know what to make for dinner" emergencies.

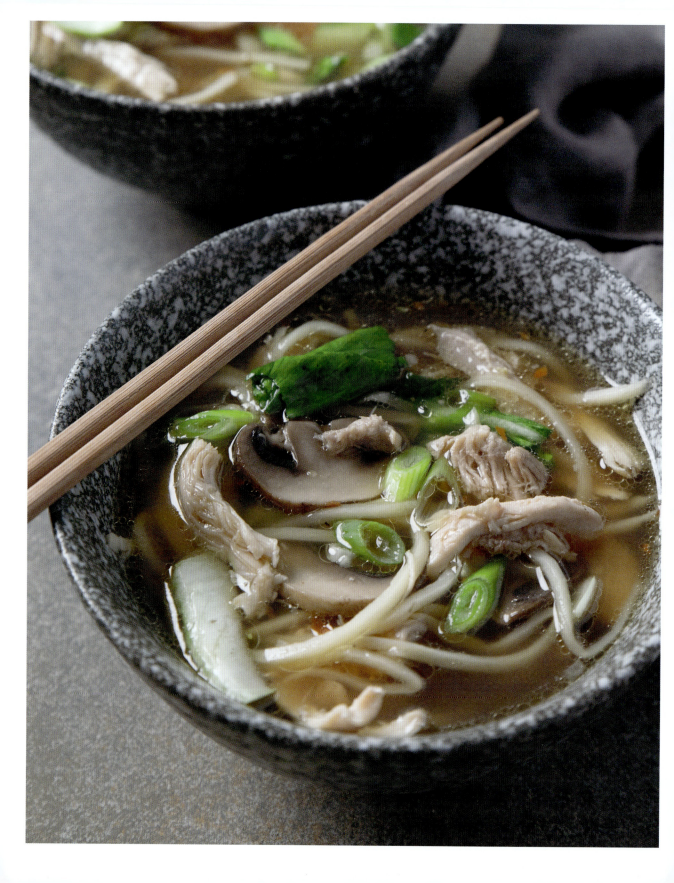

Asian Chicken Noodle Soup

Healthy and comforting, this flavorful soup is the perfect light meal when you are under the weather. The broth is full of umami as well as important electrolytes. And the light vegetables and low-carb noodles pair perfectly with shredded chicken.

Yield: 4 servings

Prep Time: 15 minutes

Cook Time: 30 minutes

Total Time: 45 minutes

EGG-FREE, DAIRY-FREE, NUT-FREE

- 1 tablespoon (15 ml) avocado oil
- 2 ounces (55 g) cremini mushrooms, sliced
- ¼ teaspoon salt
- 2 garlic cloves, minced
- 1 teaspoon minced peeled fresh ginger
- ¼ teaspoon red pepper flakes
- 3 cups (700 ml) chicken bone broth
- 2 cups (475 ml) water
- 1¼ pounds (570 g) boneless, skinless chicken thighs
- 1 head baby bok choy, chopped
- 1 package (8 ounces, or 225 g) Palmini noodles
- 1 scallion, white and light green parts, sliced
- 1 tablespoon (15 ml) tamari or soy sauce
- 1 tablespoon (15 ml) toasted sesame oil

1. In a Dutch oven or large saucepan over medium heat, heat the avocado oil until hot. Add the mushrooms, sprinkle with the salt, and sauté until they begin to brown, about 3 minutes.

2. Add the garlic, ginger, and red pepper flakes and sauté until fragrant, another minute, then pour in the bone broth and water. Bring to a boil.

3. Reduce the heat to maintain a simmer and add the chicken thighs. Cook for 20 minutes until the chicken is cooked through and no longer pink, then transfer the chicken to a plate.

4. Add the bok choy, noodles, and scallion to the pot. Shred the chicken with a fork and add it back into the soup. Stir in the tamari and sesame oil. Taste and adjust the seasoning.

5. Store any leftovers in an airtight container in the refrigerator for up to 5 days.

Low-carb noodle options

Palmini is a brand of noodles made from hearts of palm. You could also use shirataki noodles, zucchini noodles, or daikon radish noodles. If using zucchini noodles, I recommend not adding them directly to the pot. Instead, place them in individual bowls and pour the hot soup on top. This keeps them from getting overcooked and soggy.

Nutritional Information | Calories: 270 | Total Carbs: 5.3 g | Dietary Fiber: 1.8 g | Protein: 31.1 g | Fat: 14.3 g | Saturated Fat: 3.4 g

Italian Beef and Vegetable Soup

Chock-full of beefy goodness, this soup eats more like a stew. So easy to prepare, it's the perfect hearty weeknight comfort food. It freezes well too, making it a great meal prep recipe.

Yield: 6 servings

Prep Time: 15 minutes

Cook Time: 45 minutes

Total Time: 1 hour

DAIRY-FREE OPTION, EGG-FREE, NUT-FREE

2 tablespoons (28 ml) olive oil

2 ribs celery, sliced

¼ cup (40 g) chopped onion

¾ teaspoon salt

½ teaspoon ground black pepper

3 garlic cloves, minced

1 tablespoon (4 g) Italian seasoning

½ teaspoon red pepper flakes

2 pounds (910 g) ground beef

1 medium-size zucchini, halved lengthwise and sliced

6 ounces (170 g) green beans, trimmed and chopped

1 small red bell pepper, chopped

1 cup (245 g) canned diced tomatoes with their juices

4 cups (946 ml) beef broth

1 piece (1 inch, or 2.5 cm) parmesan cheese rind (optional)

1. In a large soup pot or Dutch oven over medium heat, heat the oil until hot. Add the celery and onion and sprinkle with the salt and black pepper. Sauté until the vegetables begin to soften, about 4 minutes.

2. Stir in the garlic, Italian seasoning, and red pepper flakes and continue to cook for another minute.

3. Add the ground beef to the pot and cook until nicely browned, breaking up any clumps with a wooden spoon, 8 to 10 minutes. Add the zucchini, green beans, red bell pepper, and the tomatoes and their juices and cook for 3 minutes.

4. Stir in the beef broth and add the parmesan rind (if using). Bring the pot to a simmer and cook, uncovered, for 20 minutes. Remove the parmesan rind before serving.

5. Store any leftovers in an airtight container in the refrigerator for up to 5 days or in the freezer for up to 2 months.

Tips

If you don't have a parmesan rind, skip it. It does add another depth of flavor, but it won't make or break the recipe. And if you need to be dairy-free, you will skip it anyway.

Nutritional Information | Calories: 405 | Total Carbs: 6.5 g | Dietary Fiber: 2.1 g | Protein: 31.5 g | Fat: 24 g | Saturated Fat: 9.5 g

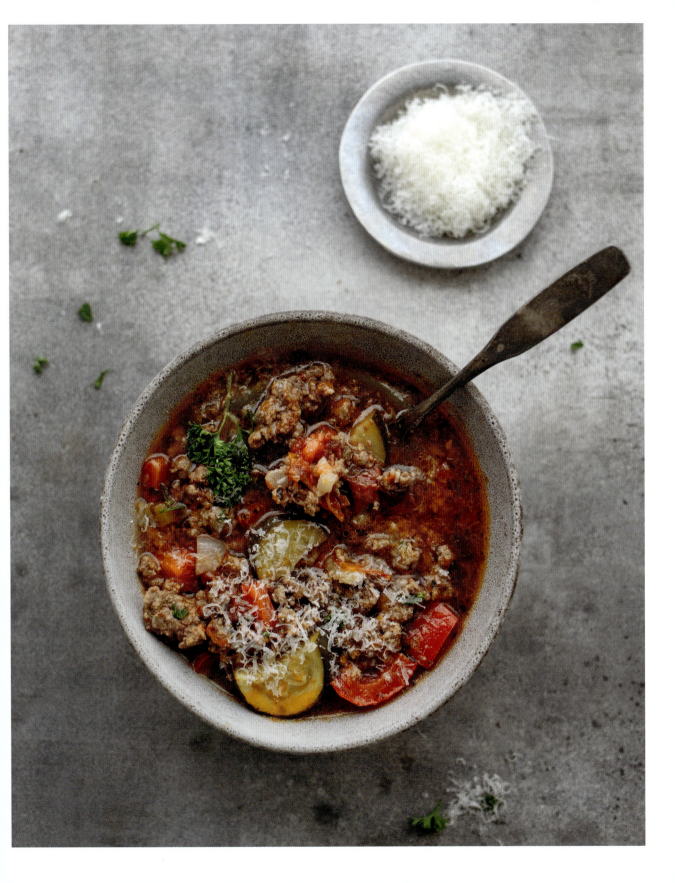

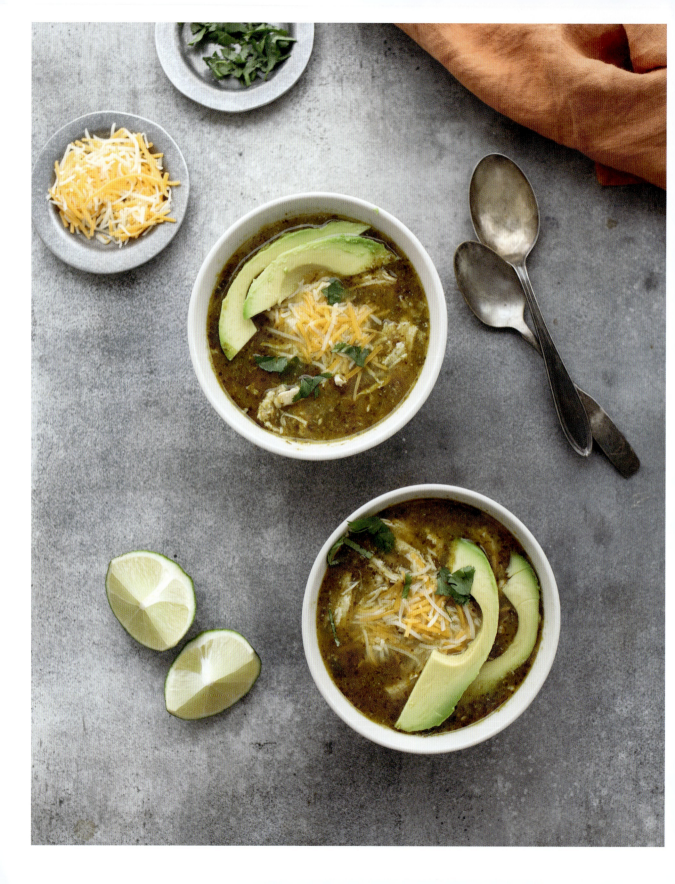

Chicken Chile Verde

If my husband had his way, I would make this easy Chicken Chile Verde every night! Serve with your favorite toppings such as shredded cheese, chopped fresh cilantro, and sour cream.

Yield: 6 servings

Prep Time: 10 minutes

Cook Time: 40 minutes

Total Time: 50 minutes

EGG-FREE, DAIRY-FREE, NUT-FREE

1 tablespoon (15 ml) olive oil

⅓ cup (55 g) chopped onion

1 large green bell pepper, chopped

1 small jalapeño pepper, minced

3 garlic cloves, minced

2 teaspoons ground cumin

¾ teaspoon dried oregano

¾ teaspoon salt

½ teaspoon ground black pepper

2 pounds (910 g) boneless, skinless chicken thighs

14 ounces (395 g) salsa verde

1 medium-size lime, cut into 6 wedges

1. In a large soup pot or Dutch oven over medium heat, heat the oil until hot. Add the onion and green bell pepper and cook until the vegetables become tender, 4 to 5 minutes. Add the jalapeño and garlic and sauté until fragrant, 1 minute more. Stir in the cumin, oregano, salt, and pepper to combine.

2. Lay the chicken thighs over the vegetables and pour in the salsa verde. Bring to a simmer and cook for 20 to 25 minutes, or until the chicken is tender and easily shredded. Transfer the chicken to a plate.

3. Use an immersion blender to blend the liquid and vegetables in the pot until mostly smooth. Alternatively, working in batches, carefully transfer the pot contents to a standard blender and blend until smooth.

4. Shred the chicken with 2 forks and return it to the pot. Stir to combine. Serve with a wedge of lime for squeezing.

5. Store any leftovers in an airtight container in the refrigerator for up to 5 days or in the freezer for up to 2 months.

Tips

- Salsa verde is a green salsa made with roasted tomatillos and green chiles. It's usually quite mild but can come in hot varieties as well.

- Remove the seeds from the jalapeño pepper or skip it if you prefer a milder dish. We like it with a kick!

Nutritional Information | Calories: 311 | Total Carbs: 7 g | Dietary Fiber: 0.7 g | Protein: 35.3 g | Fat: 12 g | Saturated Fat: 3.4 g

Creamy Tomato Sausage Soup

Up your tomato soup game with this hearty protein-packed version. Try pork, turkey, or chicken sausage. It turns out well with any of them!

Yield: 4 servings

Prep Time: 15 minutes

Cook Time: 25 minutes

Total Time: 40 minutes

EGG-FREE, NUT-FREE

1 tablespoon (15 ml) olive oil

1 pound (455 g) hot or mild bulk Italian sausage

¼ cup (40 g) chopped onion

2 garlic cloves, minced

2 cups (360 g) diced fresh tomatoes, divided

2 cups (475 ml) chicken broth

1 teaspoon dried basil or thyme

½ teaspoon salt

½ teaspoon ground black pepper

¾ cup (169 g) cottage cheese

2 ounces (55 g) cream cheese, softened

1 ounce (28 g) parmesan cheese, grated

1. In a large soup pot or Dutch oven over medium heat, heat the oil until hot. Add the sausage and cook, breaking up clumps with a wooden spoon, until nicely browned and cooked through, 8 to 10 minutes. Use a slotted spoon to transfer the sausage to a bowl, leaving the fat in the pan.

2. Add the onion and garlic to the drippings in the pan and sauté until the vegetables begin to soften, about 4 minutes.

3. Stir in 1½ cups (270 g) of the tomatoes, the broth, basil, salt, and pepper. Bring to a simmer and cook for 5 minutes.

4. In a blender or food processor, combine the cottage cheese and cream cheese. Carefully pour in the tomato/broth mixture. Blend until smooth. Return the mixture to the pot and return the sausage to the pan. Stir in the remaining ½ cup (90 g) tomatoes. Cook for a few minutes to heat through, then stir in the parmesan.

5. Store any leftovers in an airtight container in the refrigerator for up to 5 days.

Tips

If you can't find bulk sausage, use fresh links—just remove the casings before cooking.

Nutritional Information | Calories: 416 | Total Carbs: 7.3 g | Dietary Fiber: 1.3 g | Protein: 28.7 g | Fat: 27.9 g | Saturated Fat: 12.2 g

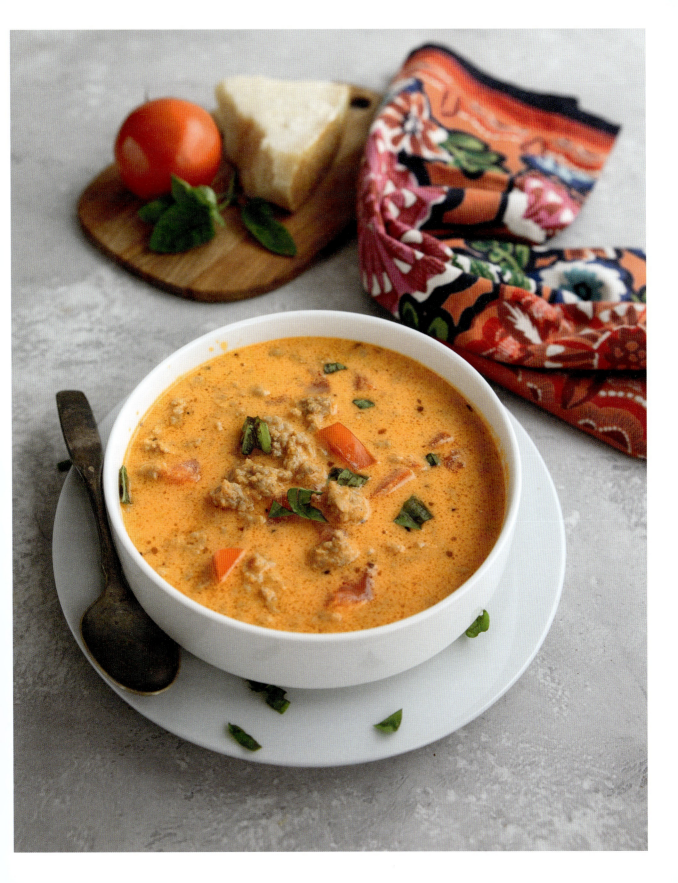

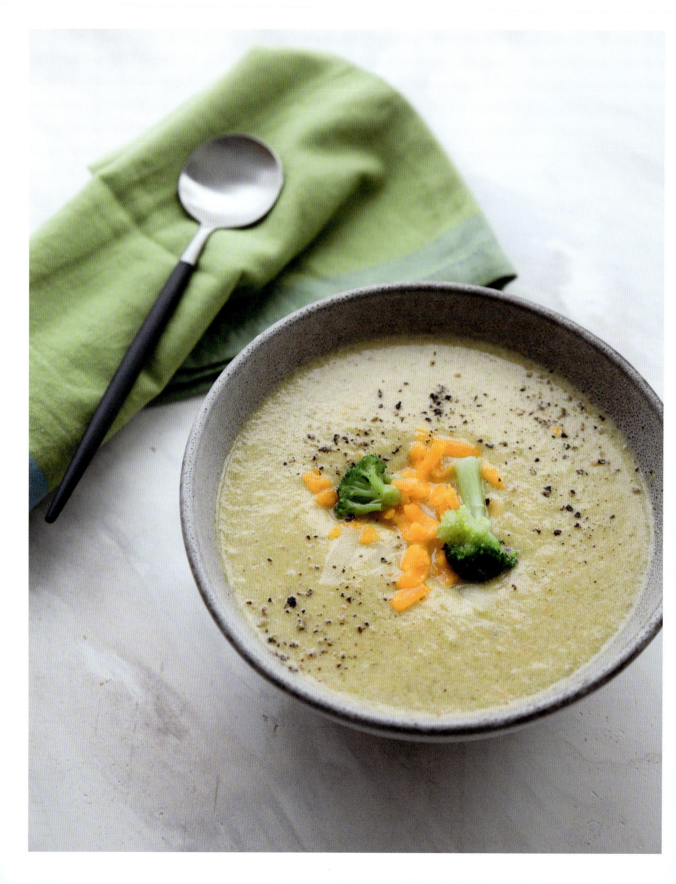

Broccoli Cheese Soup

Classic Broccoli Cheese Soup gets a protein upgrade with the help of some cottage cheese. It's extra creamy and makes a wonderful side dish or a light lunch.

Yield: 4 servings

Prep Time: 15 minutes

Cook Time: 30 minutes

Total Time: 45 minutes

EGG-FREE, NUT-FREE, VEGETARIAN OPTION

- 1 tablespoon (15 ml) olive oil
- 2 ribs celery, sliced
- ¼ cup (40 g) chopped onion
- ½ teaspoon salt
- ½ teaspoon ground black pepper
- 1 teaspoon ground cumin
- ½ teaspoon garlic powder
- ¼ teaspoon red pepper flakes
- 10 ounces (280 g) broccoli florets
- 2 cups (475 ml) chicken or vegetable broth (vegetarian option)
- 1 cup (225 g) cottage cheese
- 6 ounces (170 g) cheddar cheese, shredded

1. In a large soup pot or Dutch oven over medium heat, heat the oil until hot. Add the celery and onion and sprinkle with the salt and black pepper. Cook until the vegetables become tender, 4 to 5 minutes.

2. Add the cumin, garlic powder, and red pepper flakes and sauté for 30 seconds.

3. Stir in the broccoli and broth. Bring to a boil, then reduce the heat to maintain a simmer. Cook until the broccoli is tender, 15 to 20 minutes.

4. Stir in the cottage cheese and cheddar. Blend the soup with an immersion blender until smooth and creamy. Alternatively, carefully transfer it to a standard blender and blend, then return the soup to the pot. Taste and season as desired.

5. Store any leftovers in an airtight container in the refrigerator for up to 5 days.

Tips

When blending hot soup in a standard blender, cover the top with a kitchen towel and hold it on tightly as you blend. This reduces the chance that the lid will come off and you will be splashed with hot liquid.

Nutritional Information | Calories: 282 | Total Carbs: 8.9 g | Dietary Fiber: 2.4 g | Protein: 21.2 g | Fat: 17.1 g | Saturated Fat: 9 g

Hearty Fish Chowder

I lived in the Boston area for eleven years, so I know my chowder! And this wonderful low-carb version really delivers.

Yield: 6 servings

Prep Time: 10 minutes

Cook Time: 35 minutes

Total Time: 45 minutes

EGG-FREE, NUT-FREE

- 4 bacon slices, chopped
- ¼ cup (40 g) chopped onion
- 2 medium-size turnips, cut into ½-inch (1 cm) cubes
- 2½ cups (570 ml) chicken broth
- ½ teaspoon dried thyme
- ¾ teaspoon salt
- ½ teaspoon ground black pepper
- 1½ pounds (680 g) cod, cut into 1-inch (2.5 cm) pieces
- 1 cup (235 ml) heavy whipping cream
- 2 tablespoons (28 g) salted butter
- ¾ teaspoon glucomannan or xanthan gum (optional)

1. Line a plate with paper towels.

2. In a large saucepan over medium heat, cook the bacon until crisp, 5 to 7 minutes. With a slotted spoon, transfer the bacon to the prepared plate, leaving the grease in the pan.

3. Add the onion and turnips to the drippings and cook until the onion is tender, about 5 minutes.

4. Pour in the chicken broth, bring to a simmer, and cook until the turnips are tender, 10 to 15 minutes. Season with the thyme, salt, and pepper.

5. Add the fish and continue to simmer the chowder until the fish is cooked through and flakes easily, about 4 minutes. Stir in the heavy cream and the butter. For a thicker broth, whisk in the glucomannan (if using) at the end of cooking. Ladle into bowls and sprinkle each serving with some of the cooked bacon.

6. Store any leftovers in an airtight container in the refrigerator for up to 3 days.

Tips

Use any firm white fish for this recipe. If you crave classic clam chowder, add a 6-ounce (170 g) can of clams, undrained, in addition to the fish because clams don't have nearly as much protein on their own.

Nutritional Information | Calories: 350 | Total Carbs: 5.7 g | Dietary Fiber: 1 g | Protein: 22.7 g | Fat: 24.8 g | Saturated Fat: 14.2 g

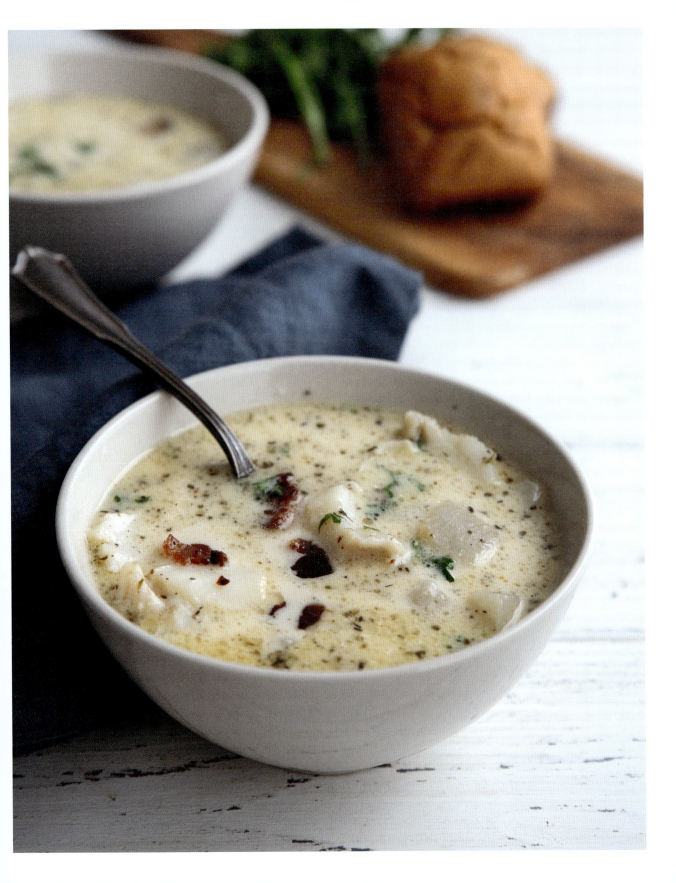

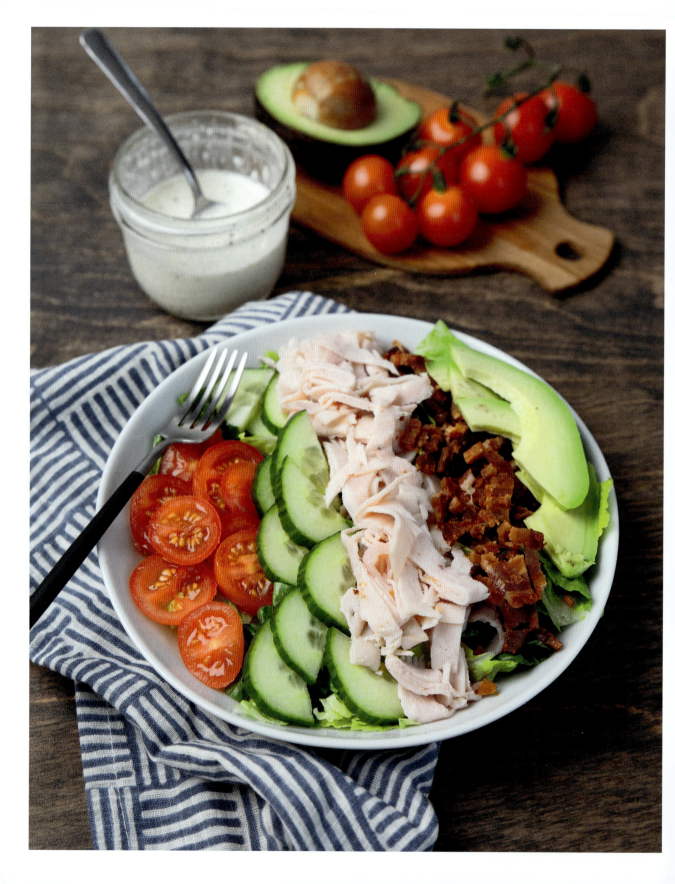

Turkey Club Salad

My favorite childhood sandwich becomes a healthier protein-packed meal. And the creamy Italian dressing is a great addition to any salad.

Yield: 4 servings

Prep Time: 15 minutes

Total Time: 15 minutes

DAIRY-FREE, NUT-FREE

FOR SALAD:

6 bacon slices, cooked to your liking

6 cups (288 g) chopped romaine lettuce

1 medium-size tomato, chopped

½ medium-size cucumber, chopped

1 medium-size avocado, peeled, pitted, and chopped

12 ounces (340 g) sliced turkey, chopped

FOR DRESSING:

3 tablespoons (42 g) mayonnaise

3 tablespoons (45 ml) apple cider vinegar

2 tablespoons (28 ml) olive oil

1 garlic clove, minced

½ teaspoon Italian seasoning

½ teaspoon salt

½ teaspoon ground black pepper

1. To make the salad: Chop the cooked bacon with a knife or crumble it with your fingers.

2. Divide the lettuce among 4 dinner plates and top each with tomato, cucumber, avocado, and turkey. Sprinkle the bacon on top.

3. To make the dressing: In a jar or bottle with a sealable lid, combine all the dressing ingredients, cover, and shake well. Serve at the table with the salad.

Tips

- You can use deli turkey slices or leftover roast turkey for this delicious salad. You could also cook some ground turkey in a skillet and let it cool.

- Use your favorite method for cooking the bacon. I like to bake it on a rimmed baking sheet at 375°F (190°C or gas mark 5) until super crisp, about 20 minutes.

Nutritional Information | Calories: 413 | Total Carbs: 8.5 g | Dietary Fiber: 4.5 g | Protein: 29.1 g | Fat: 28 g | Saturated Fat: 6 g

Blackened Chicken Caesar Salad

Yield: 4 servings

Prep Time: 20 minutes

Cook Time: 40 minutes

Total Time: 1 hour

NUT-FREE OPTION

Chicken Caesar salad gets a flavor upgrade with pan-fried blackened chicken breast. It also packs a serious nutritional punch, with 42 grams of protein and less than 8 grams of carbs per serving.

FOR CROUTONS:

1 slice Rustic Nut and Seed Bread (page 76), cubed

1 teaspoon olive oil

¼ teaspoon garlic powder

FOR DRESSING:

¼ cup (60 g) mayonnaise

1½ tablespoons (8 g) finely grated parmesan cheese

2 tablespoons (28 ml) freshly squeezed lemon juice

1 tablespoon (15 ml) olive oil

2 garlic cloves, minced

½ teaspoon cracked black pepper

Salt

FOR CHICKEN:

1 teaspoon paprika

1 teaspoon smoked paprika

1 teaspoon garlic powder

1 teaspoon onion powder

1 teaspoon salt

½ teaspoon dried oregano

½ teaspoon dried thyme

¼ teaspoon cayenne pepper

1. Preheat the oven to 250°F (120°C or gas mark ½).

2. To make the croutons: In a medium bowl, toss the bread cubes with the oil and garlic powder to coat, then spread on a baking sheet. Bake for 30 minutes, or until golden and crisp, stirring every 10 minutes or so. Let cool completely.

3. To make the dressing: In a medium bowl, whisk the mayonnaise, parmesan, lemon juice, oil, garlic, and black pepper until well combined. Taste and add salt to your liking.

4. To make the chicken: In a medium bowl, whisk all of the spices to blend.

5. Lay the breasts flat on a cutting board and carefully slice them horizontally through the middle to create 2 thinner cutlets. Rub both sides of each cutlet with the seasoning mix.

6. In a large skillet over medium-high heat, heat the oil and butter until hot and melted. Add the chicken and cook for 4 to 5 minutes per side, or until blackened and an instant-read thermometer registers 165°F (74°C) in the thickest part of the breast. Transfer to a cutting board and let rest a few minutes before slicing.

7. To make the salad: Divide the lettuce among 4 large plates and top with croutons, chicken, and shaved parmesan. Drizzle with dressing or serve at the table for everyone to dress their own salad.

Nutritional Information | Calories: 472 | Total Carbs: 7.5 g | Dietary Fiber: 3 g | Protein: 42.3 g | Fat: 23.6 g | Saturated Fat: 7.8 g

1 pound (455 g) boneless, skinless chicken breast

1 tablespoon (15 ml) olive oil

1 tablespoon (14 g) salted butter

FOR SALAD:

6 cups (288 g) chopped romaine lettuce

1 ounce (28 g) shaved or grated parmesan cheese

Tips

- All the various components can be made in advance and stored in an airtight container in the refrigerator for up to 2 days.

- Don't want to bother with the croutons but want some crunch? Try pumpkin seeds or sliced almonds instead.

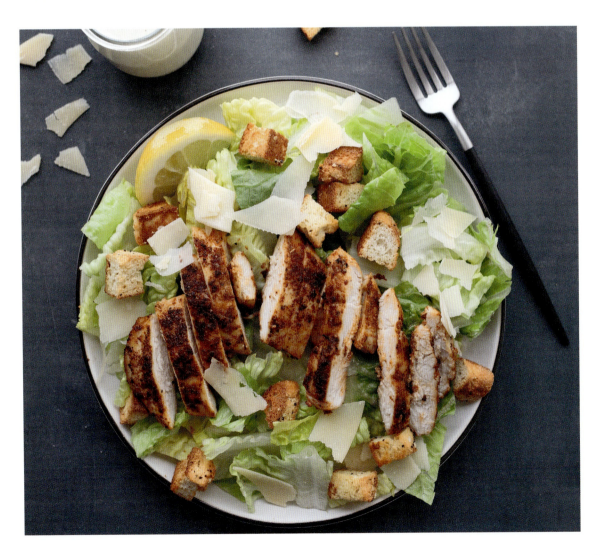

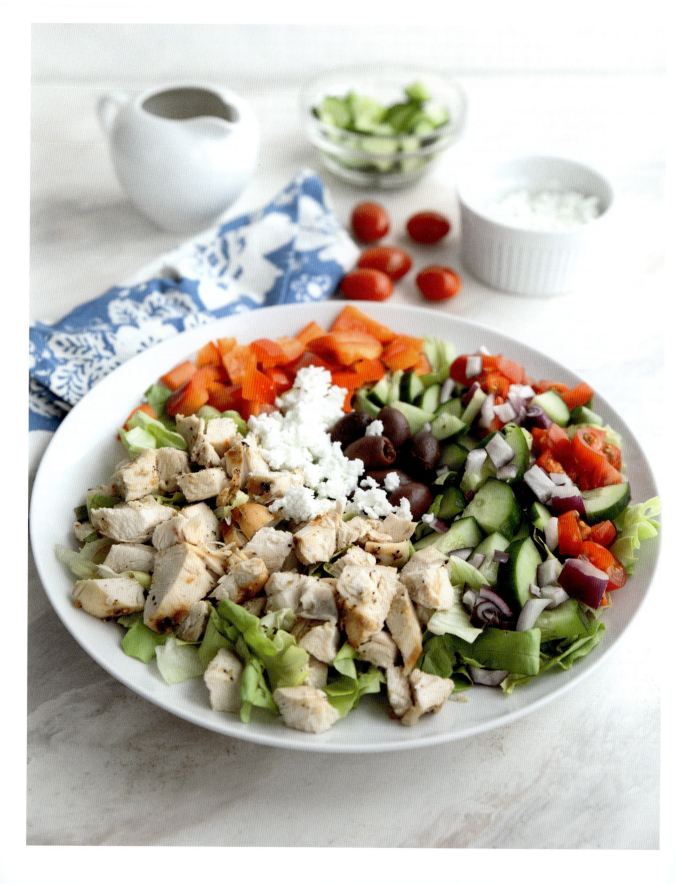

Greek Chicken Salad

This chopped Greek salad is one of my favorite summertime meals. Packed with veggies and chicken, it's bright and colorful and full of fresh flavor.

Yield: 4 servings

Prep Time: 20 minutes

Total Time: 20 minutes

EGG-FREE, NUT-FREE

FOR SALAD:

4 cups (192 g) chopped romaine lettuce

1 medium-size tomato, diced

1 small red bell pepper, diced

1 medium-size cucumber, diced

¼ cup (40 g) diced red onion

1¼ pounds (570 g) cooked chicken, chopped

½ cup (75 g) crumbled feta cheese

⅓ cup (45 g) Kalamata olives

FOR DRESSING:

¼ cup (60 ml) avocado or olive oil

¼ cup (60 ml) red wine vinegar

1 tablespoon (15 ml) freshly squeezed lemon juice

2 garlic cloves, minced

2 teaspoons Dijon mustard

½ teaspoon dried marjoram

Salt and ground black pepper

1. To make the salad: In a large bowl, toss together all the salad ingredients, then divide among 4 large plates.

2. To make the dressing: In a jar or bottle with a sealable lid, combine all the dressing ingredients, cover, and shake well. Serve at the table with the salad.

Tips

- Cook the chicken yourself or simply grab a rotisserie chicken and make it extra easy!

- For a lovely presentation, arrange the various ingredients in rows on a platter before serving.

Nutritional Information | Calories: 391 | Total Carbs: 9.8 g | Dietary Fiber: 3.3 g | Protein: 50.2 g | Fat: 23.6 g | Saturated Fat: 6.5 g

Thai Beef Salad

Steak salad has never been so flavorful. The bold flavors of lime, fish sauce, and cilantro brighten the hearty steak. It's a dinner salad you will make again and again.

Yield: 4 servings

Prep Time: 1 hour 15 minutes (includes 1 hour to marinate)

Cook Time: 10 minutes

Total Time: 1 hour 25 minutes

DAIRY-FREE, EGG-FREE, NUT-FREE

FOR MARINADE/DRESSING:

2 teaspoons grated lime zest

3 tablespoons (45 ml) freshly squeezed lime juice

2 tablespoons (28 ml) avocado oil

2 tablespoons (28 ml) fish sauce

2 tablespoons (24 g) granular sweetener

2 teaspoons sriracha

2 garlic cloves, minced

½ teaspoon ground coriander

½ teaspoon salt

FOR SALAD:

1 pound (455 g) top sirloin steak, about 1½ inches (4 cm) thick

6 cups (288 g) chopped romaine lettuce

1 medium-size cucumber, thinly sliced

1 medium-size red bell pepper, thinly sliced

¼ cup (29 g) thinly sliced red onion

2 tablespoons (2 g) fresh cilantro leaves

1 tablespoon (6 g) chopped fresh mint leaves

1. To make the marinade/dressing: In a medium-size bowl, whisk the marinade ingredients to blend.

2. To make the salad: Place the steak in a shallow dish and pour in half of the marinade, reserving the rest for dressing. Refrigerate, uncovered, to marinate for 1 hour, flipping the steak once or twice to coat.

3. Preheat a grill to medium-high heat.

4. Grill the steak over direct heat for 4 to 5 minutes per side until the internal temperature reaches 125°F to 135°F (52°C to 57°C) on an instant-read thermometer. Discard the used marinade. Alternatively, heat a skillet over medium-high heat with 1 tablespoon (15 ml) oil, then sear the steak for 4 to 5 minutes per side. Let the steak rest for 10 minutes before thinly slicing against the grain.

5. Divide the lettuce, cucumber, red bell pepper, and onion among 4 dinner plates. Top with the steak and garnish with cilantro and mint.

6. Drizzle each salad with some of the reserved dressing or pass it at the table.

Tips

Top sirloin typically has less fat than other steaks, but it's still tender enough for grilling, making it a great choice for high-protein recipes. You can also use chicken thighs or breasts in this recipe. The chicken will take longer to cook through properly on the grill, so make sure you check it with an instant-read thermometer. It should reach 165°F (74°C).

Nutritional Information | Calories: 348 | Total Carbs: 8.6 g | Dietary Fiber: 2.4 g | Protein: 33.1 g | Fat: 20.9 g | Saturated Fat: 7.4 g

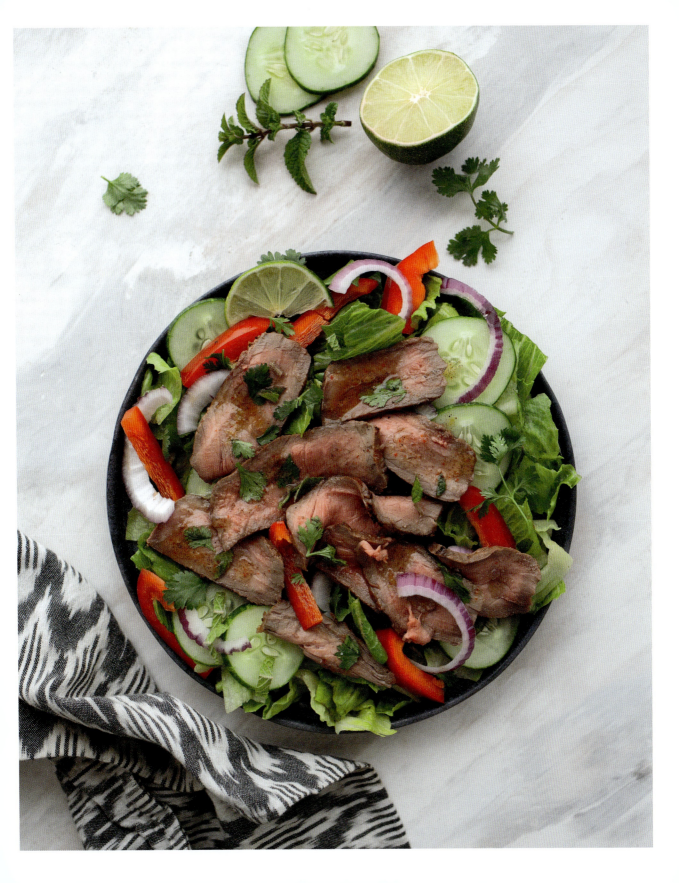

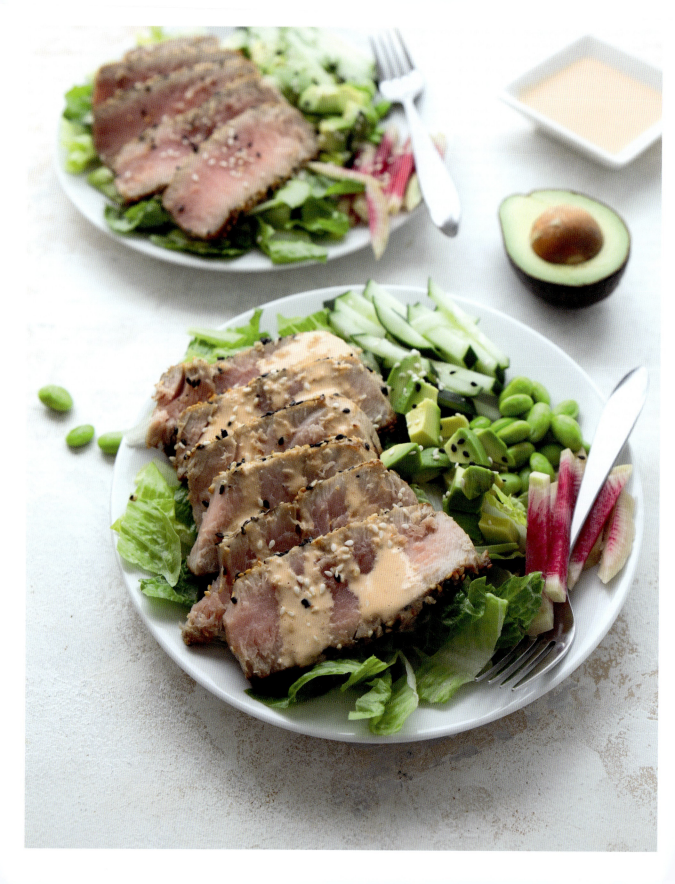

Seared Tuna Poke Salad

This salad is a great option for people who love the flavor of poke bowls but aren't comfortable eating raw fish.

Yield: 2 servings

Prep Time: 15 minutes

Cook Time: 6 minutes

Total Time: 21 minutes

DAIRY-FREE, NUT-FREE

FOR SALAD:

2 tablespoons (16 g) sesame seeds

12 ounces (340 g) ahi tuna steak (about 1 inch, or 2.5 cm, thick)

1 tablespoon (15 ml) sesame or avocado oil

2 cups (96 g) chopped romaine lettuce

¼ medium-size cucumber, cut into matchsticks

1 medium-size watermelon radish, cut into matchsticks

¼ cup (38 g) edamame beans (optional)

½ medium-size avocado, peeled and chopped

Salt

FOR DRESSING:

2 tablespoons (28 g) mayonnaise

1 tablespoon (15 ml) toasted sesame oil

1 tablespoon (15 ml) tamari or soy sauce

2 teaspoons sriracha

1. To make the salad: Spread the sesame seeds on a plate. Pat the tuna dry with paper towel and press one side into the sesame seeds to adhere. Flip the tuna over and coat the other side.

2. In a medium skillet over medium-high heat, heat the sesame oil until hot. Add the tuna and sear for 2 to 3 minutes per side. Transfer to a cutting board and let rest.

3. Divide the lettuce, cucumber, radish, edamame (if using), and avocado between 2 plates.

4. Slice the tuna with a sharp knife and layer it over the salad.

5. To make the dressing: In a medium bowl, whisk the mayonnaise, sesame oil, tamari, and sriracha to blend. Drizzle the dressing over the salads and serve.

Tips

- Cooking the tuna for 2 to 3 minutes per side yields rare to medium-rare tuna. Cook it a bit longer, if you prefer.

- Toasted sesame oil has a richer flavor than regular sesame oil and is perfect for dressings and Asian-style sauces.

Nutritional Information | Calories: 486 | Total Carbs: 9.2 g | Dietary Fiber: 5 g | Protein: 45.1 g | Fat: 28.4 g | Saturated Fat: 5 g

Buffalo Chicken Salad

This chicken salad is an easy lunch or dinner for warmer weather. The blue cheese is optional. Serve with lettuce wraps, celery sticks, or sliced cucumber. You can also use the chicken to top a green salad.

Yield: 6 servings

Prep Time: 45 minutes (includes 30 minutes to chill)

Total Time: 45 minutes

DAIRY-FREE OPTION, NUT-FREE

1½ pounds (680 g) cooked chicken breast, diced

2 ribs celery, chopped

2 scallions, white and light green parts, chopped

¼ cup (60 g) mayonnaise

¼ cup (60 ml) buffalo sauce

1 teaspoon garlic powder

½ teaspoon onion powder

Salt and ground black pepper

⅓ cup (40 g) crumbled blue cheese (optional)

1. In a large bowl, toss together the chicken, celery, and scallions to combine.

2. Add the mayonnaise, buffalo sauce, garlic powder, onion powder, and salt and pepper to taste and stir until well combined. Taste and adjust the seasoning as desired. Refrigerate until chilled, about 30 minutes.

3. To serve, top with the blue cheese (if using).

4. Store any leftovers in an airtight container in the refrigerator for up to 3 days.

Tips

Choose a plain buffalo sauce, like Frank's RedHot or Nobel Made Buffalo Sauce, as they have 0 grams of carbs per serving. Some of the "wing sauces" have added ingredients and sugar that make them higher in carbs.

Nutritional Information | Calories: 275 | Total Carbs: 1.5 g | Dietary Fiber: 0.4 g | Protein: 36.6 g | Fat: 13.1 g | Saturated Fat: 3.6 g

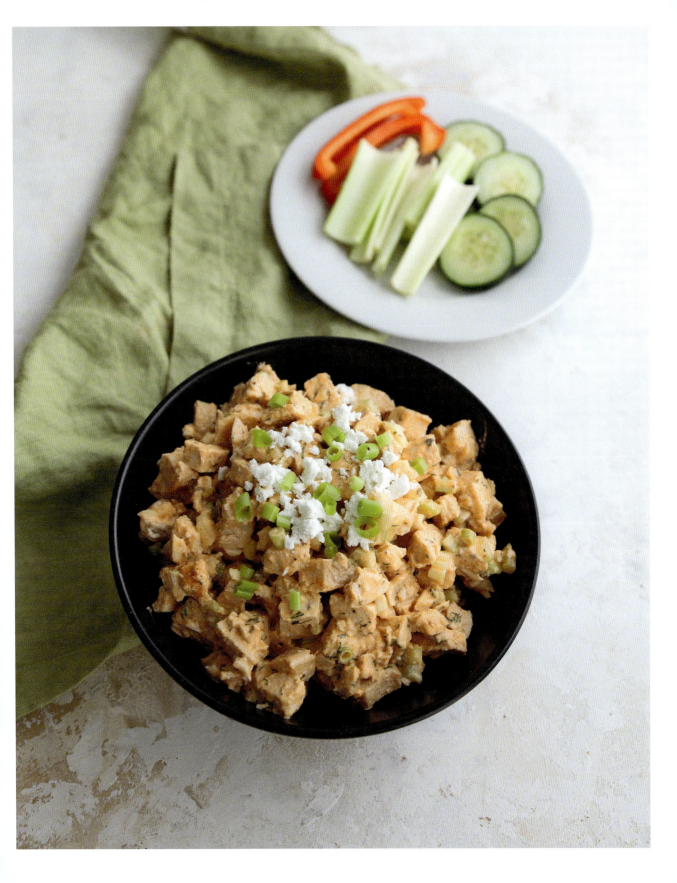

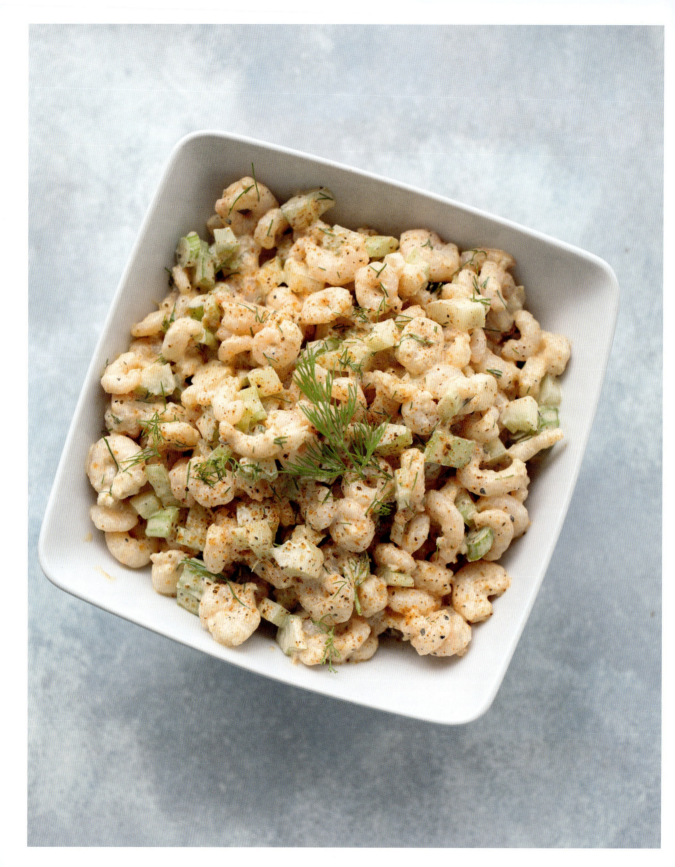

Old Bay Shrimp Salad

My family loves this deli-style shrimp salad. It's a wonderful warm-weather meal and is delicious served on toasted Easy Protein Bagels (page 75) or slices of Rustic Nut and Seed Bread (page 76).

Yield: 4 servings

Prep Time: 10 minutes

Total Time: 10 minutes

DAIRY-FREE, NUT-FREE

1 pound (455 g) small, cooked shrimp (tails removed)

3 ribs celery, chopped

1 medium-size scallion, white and light green parts, chopped

¼ cup (60 g) mayonnaise

1½ tablespoons (25 ml) freshly squeezed lemon juice

2 teaspoons Dijon mustard

1 tablespoon (4 g) chopped fresh dill

1 teaspoon Old Bay Seasoning

Salt and ground black pepper

1. In a large bowl, toss together the shrimp, celery, and scallion to combine.

2. Add the mayonnaise, lemon juice, mustard, dill, Old Bay Seasoning, and salt and pepper to taste and stir until well combined. Taste and adjust the seasonings as desired.

Tips

I like to use the tiny bay shrimp for this, which are common in my area, but you can use any cooked shrimp. If the shrimp are not on the small side, simply chop them before combining with the rest of the ingredients.

Nutritional Information | Calories: 196 | Total Carbs: 1.7 g | Dietary Fiber: 0.5 g | Protein: 23.3 g | Fat: 10.6 g | Saturated Fat: 1.8 g

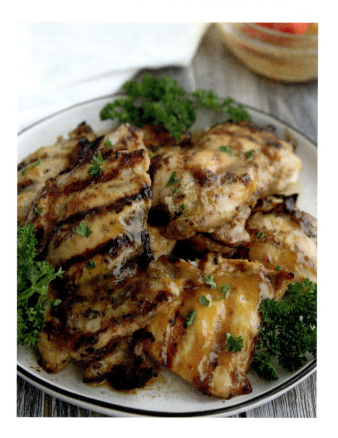

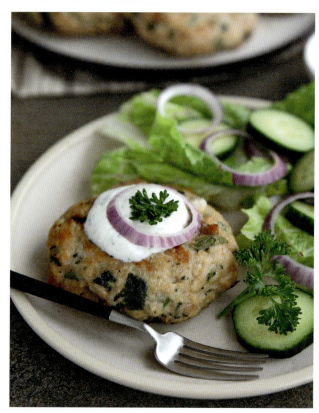

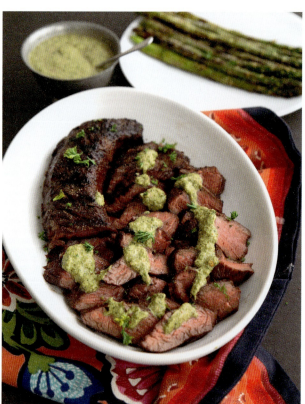

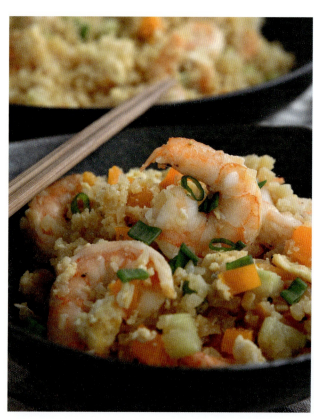

CHAPTER 8
MAIN DISHES

Most people consume plenty of protein at dinner, but it's easy to get stuck in a rut and put the same few meals on repeat. The hectic pace of modern life often means dinner is an afterthought. That's why I've crafted the recipes in this chapter to maximize flavor and minimize effort—so that even on your busiest day, you can enjoy a home-cooked, high-protein meal.

I crave variety and don't like to eat the same thing every day. I also love experimenting with different cuisines and bold flavors. In this chapter, you will find everything from classic comfort foods to takeout favorites, all with low-carb, high-protein upgrades.

In the mood for hearty Italian dishes? Try the Protein Noodle Lasagna (page 170) or the Slow Cooker Italian Pot Roast (page 169). If you crave the umami flavors of Asian-style dishes, try the Korean Beef and Broccoli (page 166) or Shrimp Fried Cauliflower Rice (page 184). And my husband highly recommends the Tex-Mex Chicken Vegetable Skillet (page 155).

Garlic Parmesan Chicken Skewers

Yield: 4 servings (2 skewers per serving)

Prep Time: 20 minutes

Cook Time: 10 minutes

Total Time: 30 minutes

EGG-FREE, NUT-FREE

My favorite flavor of wings transformed into a tasty skewer! They always turn out juicy and flavorful, whether you choose to air fry or bake them. You can even toss them on the grill! You'll need 8 skewers that can fit inside an air fryer to make this recipe.

1 pound (455 g) boneless, skinless chicken thighs

2 tablespoons (28 ml) olive oil, divided

½ teaspoon salt

½ teaspoon paprika

½ teaspoon garlic powder

½ teaspoon ground black pepper

¼ teaspoon cayenne pepper

2 tablespoons (28 g) salted butter

3 garlic cloves, finely minced

3 tablespoons (15 g) finely grated parmesan cheese

½ teaspoon dried parsley

¼ teaspoon red pepper flakes (optional)

1. If using bamboo skewers, soak them in water for at least 30 minutes before cooking.

2. Pat the chicken thighs dry and cut them into 1-inch (2.5 cm) pieces. In a large bowl, combine the chicken, 1 tablespoon (15 ml) of the oil, the salt, paprika, garlic powder, black pepper, and cayenne and toss to coat the chicken. Thread the chicken pieces onto the skewers, packing them relatively tightly to fit them all on.

3. In a microwave-safe bowl, heat the butter on high power for 15 to 20 seconds until mostly melted but not too hot. Stir in the remaining 1 tablespoon (15 ml) oil, the minced garlic, parmesan, parsley, and red pepper flakes (if using). Set aside about 2 tablespoons (28 ml) of this mixture for the finished skewers.

4. Preheat the air fryer to 400°F (200°C).

5. Arrange the skewers in a single layer in the air fryer basket and cook for 5 minutes. You may need to work in batches, depending on the size of your air fryer.

6. Remove the basket from the fryer and brush the tops of the skewers generously with the garlic-parmesan sauce. Cook for 5 minutes more, then flip and brush the second side with the sauce. Cook 1 to 2 minutes more or until the chicken reaches 165°F (74°C) on an instant-read thermometer.

7. Alternatively, preheat the oven to 425°F (220°C or gas mark 7). Set a wire rack on a rimmed baking sheet and place the skewers on the rack. Brush the tops of the

skewers generously with the garlic-parmesan sauce, then bake for
5 minutes, flip, and brush with more sauce. Bake for 5 minutes, then
broil for 1 to 2 minutes to help the chicken brown.

8. Before serving, brush the skewers with the reserved sauce.

9. Store any leftovers in an airtight container in the refrigerator for up to 5 days.

Tips

If you can't find skewers to fit in your air fryer, trim regular skewers to fit. If you
cut regular skewers in half, they are just the right size for most air fryers.

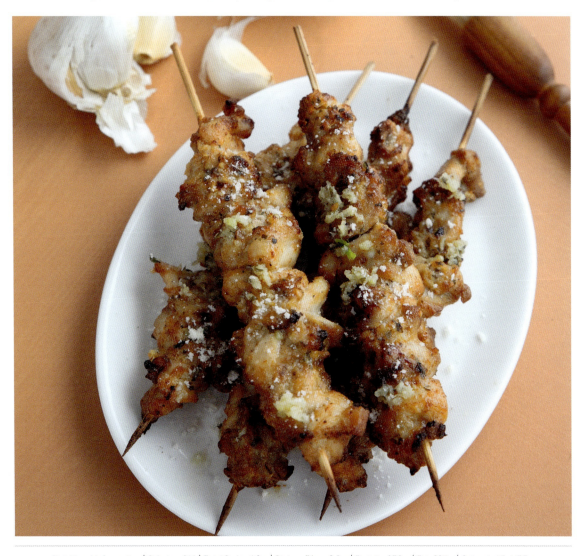

Nutritional Information | Calories: 314 | Total Carbs: 1.2 g | Dietary Fiber: 0.2 g | Protein: 27.6 g | Fat: 20.1 g | Saturated Fat: 7.5 g

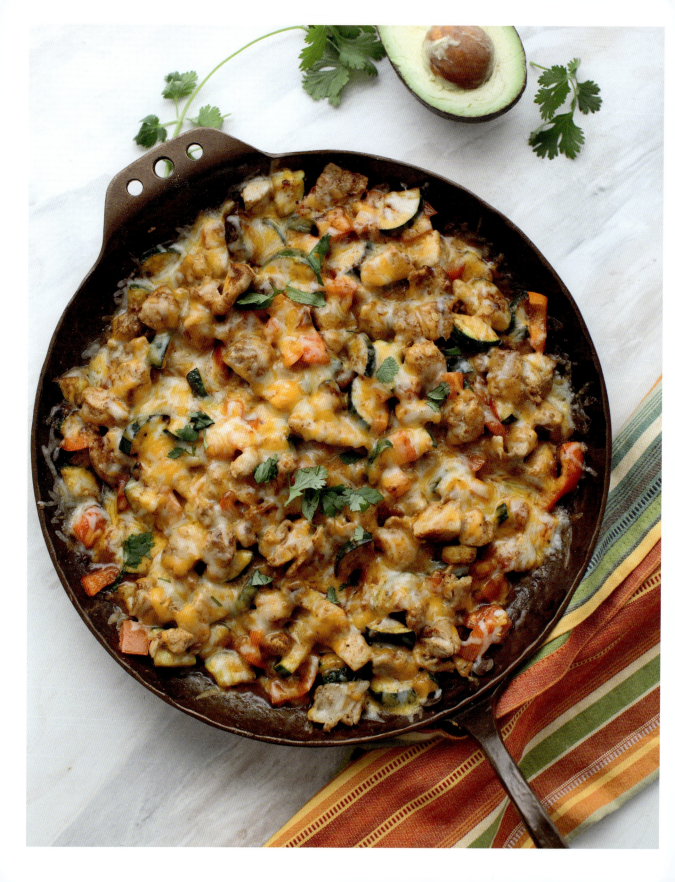

Tex-Mex Chicken Vegetable Skillet

Yield: 4 servings

Prep Time: 15 minutes

Cook Time: 20 minutes

Total Time: 35 minutes

EGG-FREE, NUT-FREE

I adore one-pan meals like this skillet, especially when they are full of flavor. This was so fragrant while cooking, my kids kept walking into the kitchen asking when dinner would be ready!

1 pound (455 g) boneless, skinless chicken thighs

Salt and ground black pepper

2 tablespoons (28 ml) olive oil, divided

1 medium-size zucchini, chopped

1 medium-size red bell pepper, chopped

3 garlic cloves, minced

2 teaspoons chili powder

1 teaspoon ground cumin

½ teaspoon chipotle powder (optional)

1 medium-size tomato, chopped

1 cup (115 g) shredded cheddar cheese

1. Pat the chicken thighs dry and cut them into ½-inch (1 cm) pieces. Season generously with salt and pepper.

2. In a large skillet over medium-high heat, heat 1 tablespoon (15 ml) of the oil until hot. Add the chicken and sauté for 5 minutes until nicely browned. Transfer to a bowl.

3. Add the remaining 1 tablespoon (15 ml) oil to the skillet. Once hot, add the zucchini, red bell pepper, and garlic. Cook, stirring frequently, until the vegetables become tender, 3 to 4 minutes.

4. Stir in the chili powder, cumin, and chipotle powder (if using) and cook until fragrant, about 1 minute. Return the chicken to the skillet, add the tomato, and toss to combine. Taste and add more salt and pepper as desired.

5. Spread the mixture evenly in the skillet and sprinkle it with the cheese. Cover and cook until bubbly and the cheese is melted, 8 to 10 minutes.

6. Store any leftovers in an airtight container in the refrigerator for up to 5 days.

Tips

This is a full meal in a pan with protein and veggies, so you can just scoop it into a bowl and eat as is. Or serve it over cauliflower rice for even more nutrition. Garnish with your favorite toppings, like avocado or chopped fresh cilantro.

Nutritional Information | Calories: 391 | Total Carbs: 6.5 g | Dietary Fiber: 2.1 g | Protein: 34.5 g | Fat: 22.5 g | Saturated Fat: 8.8 g

Honey Mustard Chicken Thighs

These Honey Mustard Chicken Thighs are a low-carb dinnertime win. They have a sweet, tangy marinade that no one would guess is totally sugar-free. I must have made this at least ten times this past summer!

Yield: 4 servings

Prep Time: 2 hours 5 minutes (includes 2 hours to marinate)

Cook Time: 15 minutes

Total Time: 2 hours 20 minutes

DAIRY-FREE, EGG-FREE, NUT-FREE

¼ cup (60 g) Dijon mustard

¼ cup (80 g) allulose honey alternative

1 tablespoon (15 ml) olive oil, plus more for the grill

1 teaspoon garlic powder

¾ teaspoon salt

½ teaspoon ground black pepper

¼ teaspoon cayenne pepper

1¼ pounds (570 g) boneless, skinless chicken thighs

1. In a medium bowl, whisk the mustard, allulose honey, oil, garlic powder, salt, black pepper, and cayenne to combine.

2. Place the chicken thighs in a large bowl. Pour about half of the honey mustard over the chicken and toss to coat. Reserve the remaining sauce. Refrigerate the chicken, uncovered, to marinate for 1 to 2 hours.

3. Preheat a grill to medium-high heat and brush the grates lightly with oil.

4. Grill the chicken over direct heat until the center reaches 165°F (74°C) on an instant-read thermometer, 6 to 7 minutes per side. Brush with a little of the reserved honey mustard sauce and grill for another minute or so. Alternatively, bake the thighs in the oven at 375°F (190°C or gas mark 5) for about 20 minutes until the center reaches 165°F (74°C) on an instant-read thermometer. Transfer to a plate and brush with more sauce, as desired.

5. Store any leftovers in an airtight container in the refrigerator for up to 5 days.

Tips

Allulose honey is just liquid allulose with honey flavors. I like the one from All-u-Lose. You can also use 3 tablespoons (36 g) brown sugar substitute mixed with 2 teaspoons water.

Nutritional Information | Calories: 275 | Total Carbs: 1.2 g | Dietary Fiber: 0 g | Protein: 33.3 g | Fat: 12.9 g | Saturated Fat: 3.4 g

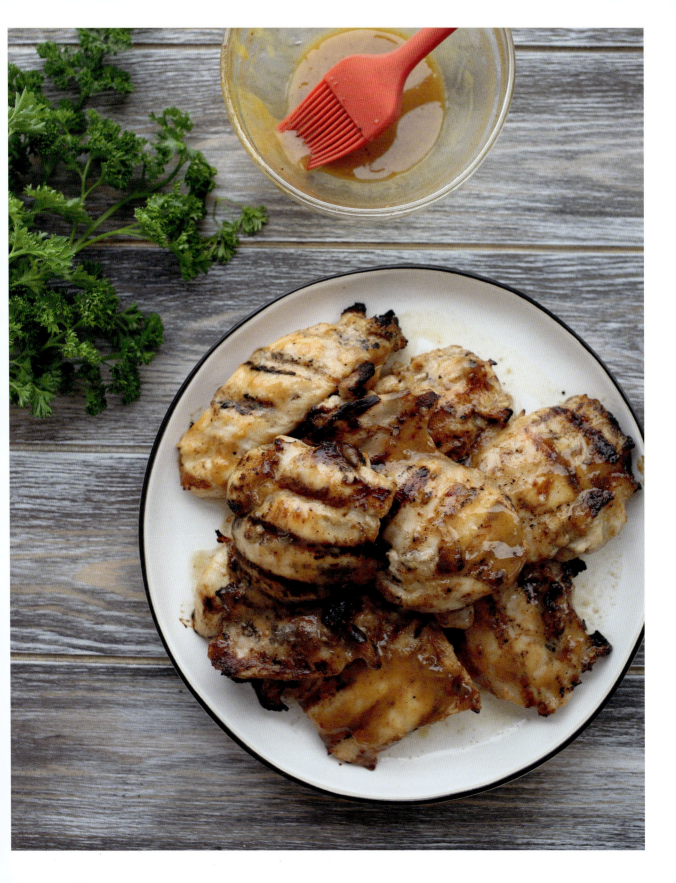

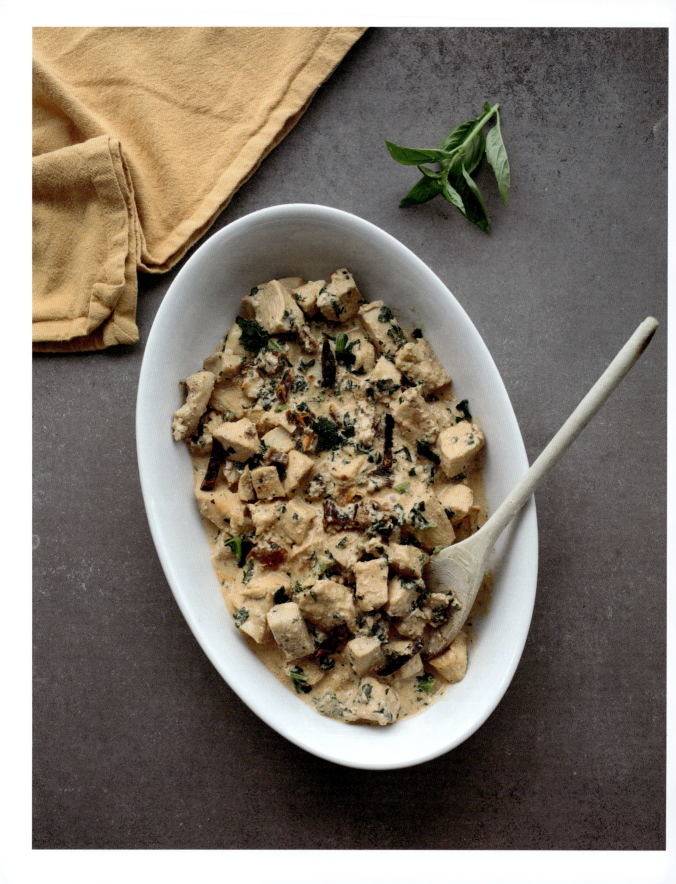

Slow Cooker Tuscan Chicken

Yield: 6 servings

Prep Time: 15 minutes

Cook Time: 6 hours

Total Time: 6 hours 15 minutes

EGG-FREE, NUT-FREE

This is what I like to call a "dump-and-run" recipe. You simply dump everything into the pot and walk away. Let your slow cooker do the cooking for you! Serve over cauliflower rice or zucchini noodles.

1½ pounds (680 g) boneless, skinless chicken breast, cut into bite-size pieces

4 ounces (115 g) cream cheese, softened, cut into 8 pieces

½ cup (120 ml) heavy whipping cream

½ cup (120 ml) chicken broth

6 ounces (170 g) chopped spinach

⅓ cup (40 g) chopped sun-dried tomatoes

4 garlic cloves, minced

1 teaspoon Italian seasoning

¾ teaspoon salt

½ teaspoon ground black pepper

¼ teaspoon red pepper flakes

1 tablespoon (16 g) tomato paste

1 ounce (28 g) grated parmesan cheese

1. Lightly grease the ceramic insert of a 5- to 6-quart (4.7 to 5.7 L) slow cooker.

2. Spread the chicken on the bottom of the pot and top with the cream cheese, cream, broth, spinach, sun-dried tomatoes, garlic, Italian seasoning, salt, black pepper, and red pepper flakes. Cover and cook on low for 6 hours.

3. Add the tomato paste and parmesan and stir until the sauce is creamy and smooth. Serve hot.

4. Store any leftovers in an airtight container in the refrigerator for up to 5 days.

Tips
Chicken breasts tend to be large and can weigh as much as 10 ounces (280 g). I prefer to chop them up for this recipe so they can be divided into appropriate servings more easily. You could also use boneless, skinless chicken thighs and leave them whole or chop them up.

Nutritional Information | Calories: 344 | Total Carbs: 5.7 g | Dietary Fiber: 1.2 g | Protein: 39.6 g | Fat: 17.2 g | Saturated Fat: 10.2 g

Spinach Feta Chicken Burgers

These are the best chicken burgers I have ever made, and I don't say that lightly. They hold together nicely without any filler and have wonderful flavor. See top right of page 150 for photo.

Yield: 6 large burgers
(1 burger per serving)

Prep Time: 1 hour 20 minutes
(includes 1 hour to chill)

Cook Time: 18 minutes

Total Time: 1 hours 38 minutes

EGG-FREE, NUT-FREE

FOR BURGERS:

8 ounces (225 g) frozen spinach, thawed and squeezed of excess moisture

½ cup (75 g) crumbled feta cheese

1 tablespoon (4 g) chopped fresh parsley

3 garlic cloves, minced

1 teaspoon salt

½ teaspoon ground black pepper

½ teaspoon ground cumin

2 pounds (910 g) ground chicken

FOR GARLIC DILL SAUCE:

½ cup (120 g) plain Greek yogurt

1 tablespoon (15 ml) freshly squeezed lemon juice

1 garlic clove, minced

¾ teaspoon dried dill

¼ teaspoon salt

¼ teaspoon ground black pepper

1. To make the burgers: Line a plate with wax paper. In a large bowl, whisk the spinach, feta, parsley, garlic, salt, pepper, and cumin to combine. Add the ground chicken and mix well with your hands. Form the mixture into 6 patties about ¾ inch (2 cm) thick and place them on the prepared plate. Refrigerate for 1 hour.

2. Preheat a grill to medium-high heat and brush the grates with oil.

3. Carefully lay the burgers on the grates over direct heat and cook for 7 to 9 minutes per side, or until the center reaches 165°F (74°C) on an instant-read thermometer. Alternatively, in a large skillet over medium heat, heat 2 tablespoons (28 ml) oil until hot. Cook the burgers for 6 to 7 minutes per side until they reach 165°F (74°C) on an instant-read thermometer. Transfer to a plate.

4. To make the sauce: In a medium-size bowl, whisk all the sauce ingredients until well blended. Serve at the table with the burgers.

5. Store any leftovers in an airtight container in the refrigerator for up to 5 days.

Tips

I find that if the burgers are flavorful enough, you don't need a bun. These are great with just a salad and some sauce on top.

Nutritional Information | Calories: 276 | Total Carbs: 4 g | Dietary Fiber: 1.2 g | Protein: 30.4 g | Fat: 14.4 g | Saturated Fat: 5.8 g

Turkey Pojarski

"Pojarski" is a Russian dish made with chopped or minced meat. I have no idea how my husband's family came by this recipe, but they often made it when he was a kid. I modified it for a low-carb version, and it has become a family favorite for us too.

Yield: 6 patties (1 patty per serving)

Prep Time: 50 minutes (includes 30 minutes to chill)

Cook Time: 20 minutes

Total Time: 1 hours 10 minutes

EGG-FREE, NUT-FREE OPTION

2 pounds (910 g) ground turkey

⅔ cup (75 g) almond flour

½ cup (30 g) chopped fresh parsley

1 teaspoon ground cumin

Salt and ground black pepper

¼ cup (60 ml) olive oil, divided

8 ounces (225 g) cremini mushrooms, sliced

¼ cup (40 g) chopped onion

⅓ cup (80 ml) chicken broth

½ cup (115 g) sour cream

1. Line a plate with wax paper. In a large mixing bowl, combine the ground turkey, almond flour, parsley, cumin, 1 teaspoon salt, and ½ teaspoon pepper. Mix by hand until well combined. Form the mixture into 6 large patties, about 1 inch (2.5 cm) thick, and place on the prepared plate. Refrigerate for 30 minutes to firm up.

2. In a large skillet over medium heat, heat 2 tablespoons (28 ml) of the oil until hot. Add the patties to the skillet and cook for 6 to 7 minutes per side until the centers reach 165°F (74°C) on an instant-read thermometer. Transfer to a plate.

3. Add the remaining 2 tablespoons (28 ml) oil to the pan. Once hot, add the mushrooms and onion and sprinkle with a little salt and pepper. Sauté until the mushrooms are golden brown, about 4 minutes.

4. Pour in the broth and bring just to a simmer. Remove from the heat and stir in the sour cream until smooth and well combined. Serve the patties with the sauce over the top.

5. Store any leftovers in an airtight container in the refrigerator for up to 5 days.

Tips

- Don't skip the chilling time—it helps the patties hold together better when frying them.

- Use pumpkin seed meal or sunflower seed meal instead of almond flour for a nut-free version.

Nutritional Information | Calories: 428 | Total Carbs: 6 g | Dietary Fiber: 1.9 g | Protein: 32.8 g | Fat: 29.8 g | Saturated Fat: 7.2 g

Hanger Steak with Chimichurri

Hanger steak has become one of my favorite cuts of beef. It's extremely tender but has much less fat than other steaks, which makes it perfect for a high-protein dinner. Served with a tangy chimichurri, it makes an easy but elegant meal for family or guests.

Yield: 6 servings

Prep Time: 15 minutes

Cook Time: 15 minutes

Total Time: 30 minutes

DAIRY-FREE, EGG-FREE, NUT-FREE

FOR CHIMICHURRI:

- 1½ cups (90 g) fresh parsley leaves
- ¼ cup (40 g) chopped red onion
- 2 garlic cloves, peeled
- ¼ cup (60 ml) red wine vinegar
- 3 tablespoons (45 ml) olive oil
- ½ teaspoon salt
- ½ teaspoon ground black pepper
- ¼ teaspoon red pepper flakes

FOR STEAK:

- 2 pounds (910 g) hanger steak
- ¾ teaspoon salt
- ½ teaspoon ground black pepper

1. To make the chimichurri: In a blender or food processor, combine all of the chimichurri ingredients. Blend until smooth or leave the sauce a little chunky.

2. To make the steak: Preheat a grill to medium-high heat.

3. Season the steak all over with salt and black pepper. Place the steak on the grill over direct heat and cook for 5 to 7 minutes per side until the internal temperature reaches 125°F (52°C) on an instant-read thermometer for medium-rare. Alternatively, in a large skillet over medium-high heat, heat 1 tablespoon (15 ml) avocado oil. Add the steak and cook, turning frequently, until the internal temperature reaches 125°F (52°C) for medium-rare.

4. Transfer to a platter and let rest for 5 minutes before slicing against the grain. Serve with the chimichurri spooned over the steak or on the side.

5. Store any leftovers in an airtight container in the refrigerator for up to 5 days.

Tips

Hanger steak is so tender, you don't have to worry about slicing it thinly for serving. I usually cut it into ½-inch (1 cm) slices.

Nutritional Information | Calories: 389 | Total Carbs: 1.9 g | Dietary Fiber: 0.6 g | Protein: 46.7 g | Fat: 18.9 g | Saturated Fat: 6.3 g

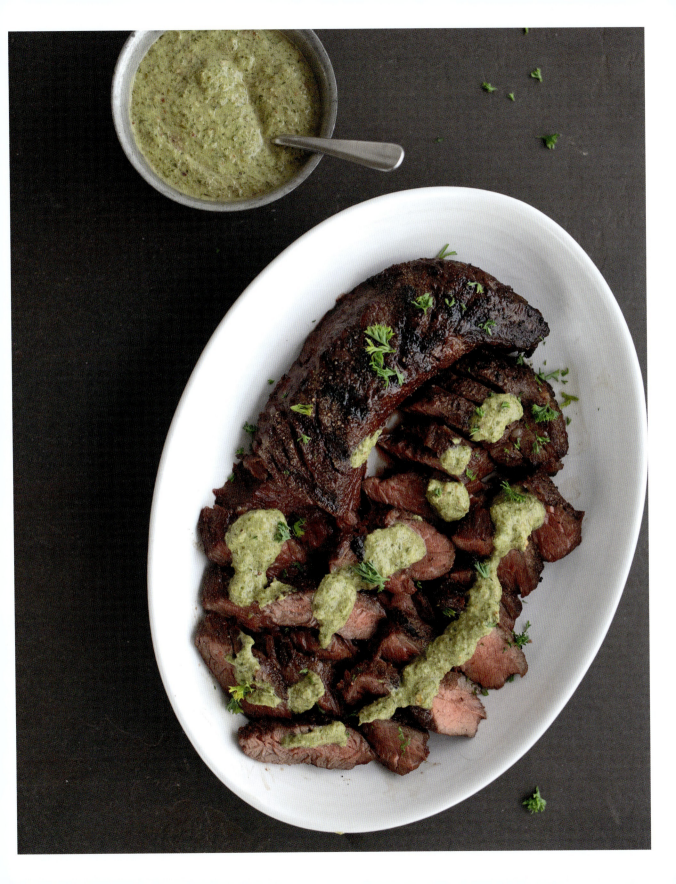

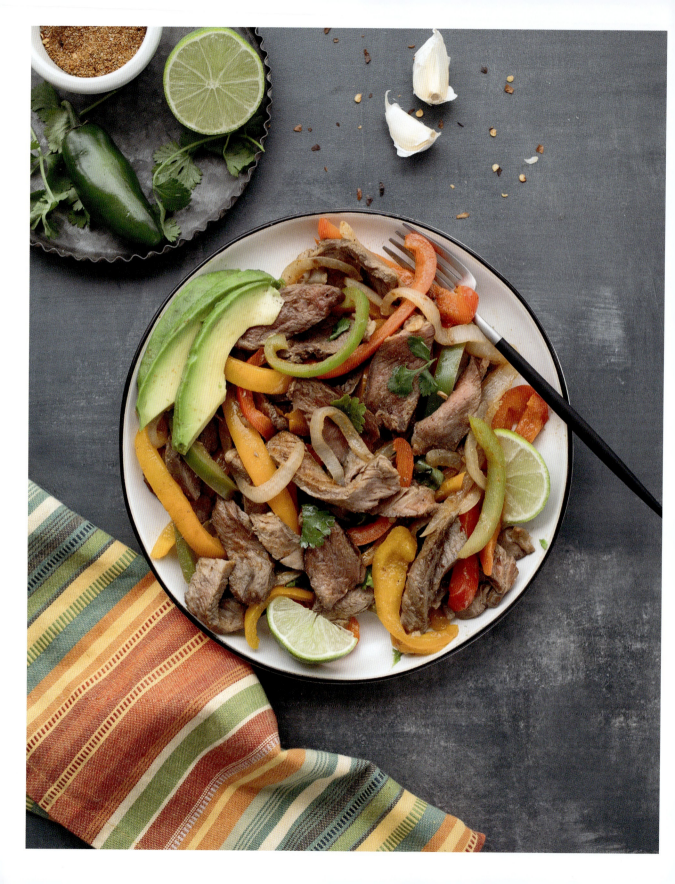

Easy Steak Fajitas

Fajitas are quite low carb as long as you don't load up on the rice and beans! Serve these with Egg White Wraps (page 84) if you're craving tortillas. My favorite way to eat this is in a big bowl with cauliflower rice and guacamole. It also makes a fabulous salad topping.

Yield: 4 servings

Prep Time: 2 hour 20 minutes (includes 2 hours to marinate)

Cook Time: 15 minutes

Total Time: 2 hours 35 minutes

DAIRY-FREE, EGG-FREE, NUT-FREE

FOR MARINADE:

2 tablespoons (28 ml) freshly squeezed lime juice

2 tablespoons (28 ml) olive oil

2 tablespoons (28 ml) water

3 garlic cloves, minced

2 teaspoons smoked paprika

1 teaspoon onion powder

¾ teaspoon chipotle powder, or 1½ teaspoons chili powder

½ teaspoon ground cumin

½ teaspoon salt

½ teaspoon ground black pepper

FOR FAJITAS:

1 pound (455 g) flank steak, thinly sliced

1 tablespoon (15 ml) olive oil

1 medium-size green bell pepper, thinly sliced

½ medium-size red bell pepper, thinly sliced

½ orange or yellow bell pepper, thinly sliced

⅓ medium-size onion, thinly sliced

2 tablespoons (2 g) chopped fresh cilantro

1. To make the marinade: In a large bowl, whisk all of the marinade ingredients to combine.

2. To make the fajitas: Add the sliced steak to the marinade and toss to combine. Refrigerate, uncovered, to marinate for at least 2 hours.

3. Drain the steak from the marinade. Discard the used marinade.

4. Heat a large skillet over medium-high heat. Add the steak to the hot skillet and sauté until nicely browned on the outside and still a little pink in the middle, about 5 minutes. Transfer to a bowl.

5. Remove any juices from the pan and pour in the oil. Once hot, add the bell peppers and onion and sauté until just tender, about 5 minutes.

6. Return the steak slices to the pan and toss to warm through. Sprinkle with cilantro and serve hot.

7. Store any leftovers in an airtight container in the refrigerator for up to 5 days.

Tips

The marinated meat can release a lot of liquid when it hits the hot pan. Removing the excess liquid before you add the veggies lets you sauté them until they are crisp-tender, rather than stewing them.

Nutritional Information | Calories: 295 | Total Carbs: 6.9 g | Dietary Fiber: 2.1 g | Protein: 25.2 g | Fat: 17.2 g | Saturated Fat: 4.8 g

Korean Beef and Broccoli

This quick-and-easy dinner recipe relies on ground beef and frozen broccoli. It's simple enough to whip up on a weeknight. And the leftovers make a fabulous lunch the next day.

Yield: 4 servings

Prep Time: 5 minutes

Cook Time: 15 minutes

Total Time: 20 minutes

DAIRY-FREE, EGG-FREE, NUT-FREE

FOR SAUCE:

¼ cup (60 ml) tamari or soy sauce

¼ cup (48 g) granular sweetener

1 tablespoon (15 ml) sesame oil

2 teaspoons grated peeled fresh ginger

2 garlic cloves, minced

¼ teaspoon red pepper flakes

¼ teaspoon hot sauce (optional)

FOR BEEF AND BROCCOLI:

1 tablespoon (15 ml) avocado oil

1¼ pounds (570 g) ground beef

1 medium-size scallion, white and green parts, sliced

12 ounces (340 g) frozen broccoli, thawed

1 teaspoon toasted sesame seeds

1. To make the sauce: In a glass measuring cup or a small bowl, whisk the tamari, sweetener, sesame oil, ginger, garlic, red pepper flakes, and hot sauce (if using) to blend.

2. To make the beef and broccoli: In a large skillet over medium heat, heat the avocado oil until hot. Add the ground beef and stir-fry until no pink remains, about 7 minutes, breaking up any clumps.

3. Stir in the sauce and scallion and cook until the sauce has reduced and thickened, 2 to 3 minutes.

4. Add the thawed broccoli, toss to combine, and cook for 2 to 3 minutes to heat through. Garnish with sesame seeds before serving.

5. Store any leftovers in an airtight container in the refrigerator for up to 5 days.

Tips

- Tamari is a slightly more flavorful version of soy sauce that is gluten-free. I prefer it for my low-carb recipes.

- I like to use frozen broccoli, as it requires no precooking. If you use fresh, steam it until it is fork-tender before adding it to the beef.

- You can also make this dish with ground chicken or turkey.

How to toast sesame seeds

If you can't find them already toasted, spread the sesame seeds in a skillet over medium heat. Cook, stirring almost constantly, until they are lightly browned. Remove them from the pan immediately.

Nutritional Information | Calories: 408 | Total Carbs: 7.3 g | Dietary Fiber: 2.5 g | Protein: 30.2 g | Fat: 24.6 g | Saturated Fat: 9.1 g

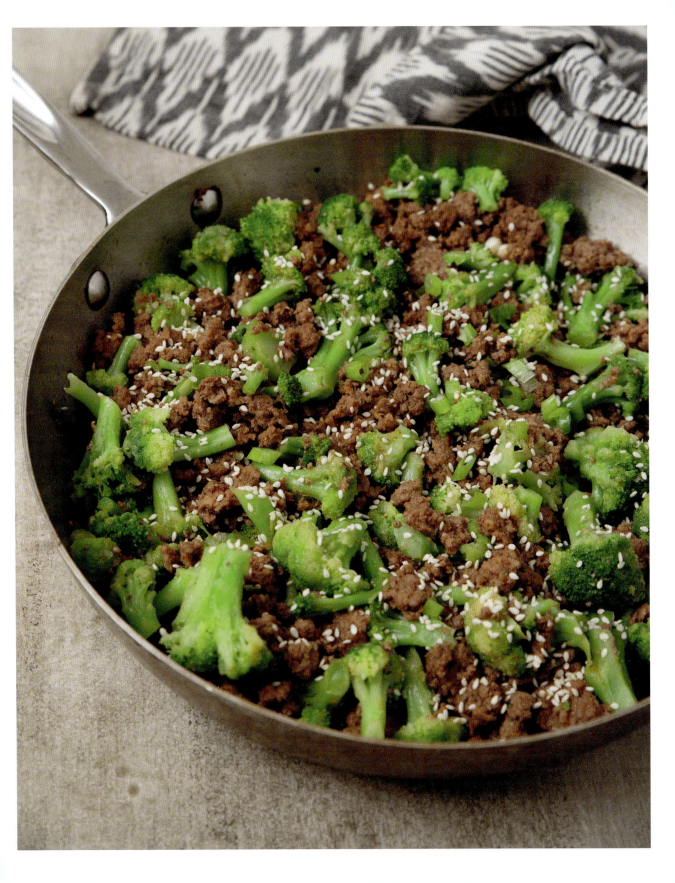

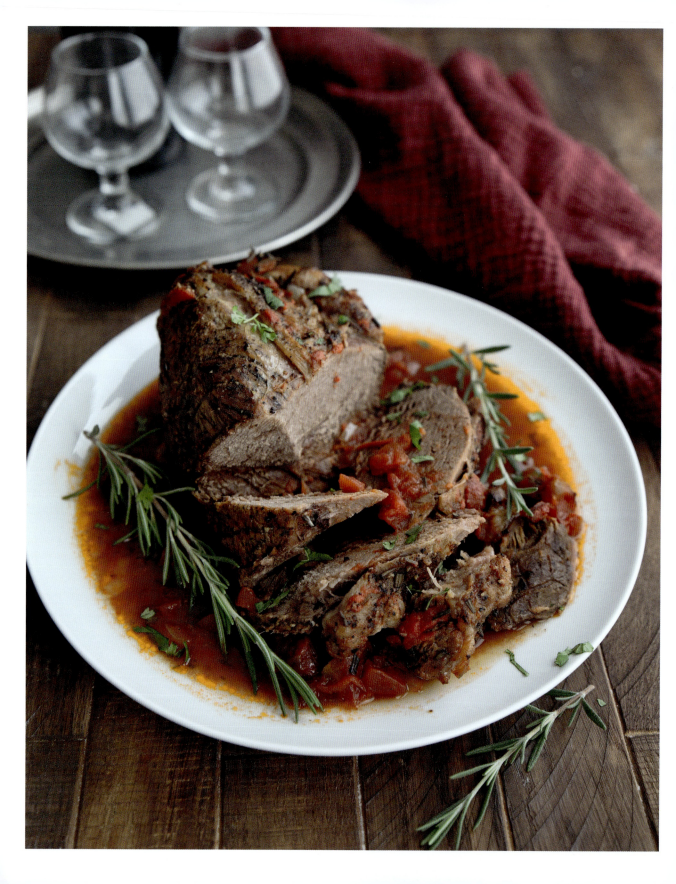

Slow Cooker Italian Pot Roast

Hearty beef is slow cooked in a flavorful tomato sauce until it becomes melt-in-your-mouth tender. With very little prep time, you can start this recipe in the morning and come home to a perfectly comforting meal. This makes plenty of sauce, so it's wonderful served over mashed cauliflower or your favorite low-carb noodles.

Yield: 8 servings

Prep Time: 10 minutes

Cook Time: 8 hours

Total Time: 8 hours 10 minutes

DAIRY-FREE, EGG-FREE, NUT-FREE

3 pounds (1.4 kg) beef chuck roast

Salt and ground black pepper

1 tablespoon (15 ml) olive oil

1½ cups (368 g) canned diced tomatoes with their juices

½ cup (120 ml) red wine or beef broth

¼ cup (40 g) chopped onion

3 garlic cloves, minced

1 tablespoon (2 g) chopped fresh rosemary leaves

2 bay leaves

¼ teaspoon red pepper flakes

1. Pat the roast dry with paper towel and season it all over with salt and black pepper.

2. In a large skillet over medium-high heat, heat the oil until hot. Add the roast and brown on all sides, about 6 minutes. Place the roast in the bottom of a 5- to 6-quart (4.8 to 5.7 L) slow cooker.

3. Add the tomatoes and their juices, red wine, onion, garlic, rosemary, bay leaves, red pepper flakes, and a little more salt and black pepper. Cover and cook on low for 6 to 8 hours until the beef is tender and easily pierced with a fork. Transfer the beef to a cutting board and slice or shred, as desired.

4. Remove the bay leaves, stir the sauce in the slow cooker, and serve over the roast.

5. Store any leftovers in an airtight container in the refrigerator for up to 5 days.

Tips

Choose a chuck roast with at least a little fat for flavor and tenderness. Browning the beef on all sides before slow cooking helps bring out the best flavors.

Nutritional Information | Calories: 376 | Total Carbs: 3.8 g | Dietary Fiber: 0.7 g | Protein: 33.1 g | Fat: 24.3 g | Saturated Fat: 10 g

Protein Noodle Lasagna

Who needs pasta when you've got high-protein egg white wraps? Turns out they make perfect layers for a healthy lasagna.

Yield: 10 servings

Prep Time: 30 minutes

Cook Time: 40 minutes

Total Time: 1 hour 10 minutes (not including the time to make the egg white wraps)

NUT-FREE

1½ pounds (680 g) ground beef or ground turkey

1 teaspoon salt, divided

½ teaspoon ground black pepper

¼ teaspoon red pepper flakes

1½ cups (375 g) canned puréed tomatoes

15 ounces (425 g) full-fat ricotta cheese

6 ounces (170 g) frozen spinach, thawed and squeezed of excess moisture

½ cup (50 g) grated parmesan cheese

1 large egg

2 garlic cloves, minced

1½ teaspoons olive oil, plus more for brushing

6 to 8 Egg White Wraps (page 84)

8 ounces (225 g) shredded mozzarella cheese

1. Heat a large sauté pan or skillet over medium heat. Add the ground beef and cook for 7 to 10 minutes, breaking up any clumps with the back of a wooden spoon, until cooked through. Sprinkle with ¾ teaspoon of the salt, the black pepper, and red pepper flakes. Stir in the tomatoes.

2. In a large bowl, stir together the ricotta, spinach, parmesan, egg, garlic, and the remaining ¼ teaspoon salt to combine.

3. Preheat the oven to 350°F (180°C or gas mark 4) and brush a 9 × 13-inch (23 × 33 cm) glass or ceramic baking dish with oil.

4. Lay 2 egg white wraps in the bottom of the prepared pan, cutting to fit. Use extra egg white wraps as needed. You don't need to cover the whole bottom perfectly!

5. Spread one-third of the ricotta mixture over the wraps, then one-third of the meat sauce, and one-quarter of the mozzarella. Repeat these layers 2 more times, finishing with mozzarella.

6. Bake for 30 minutes until bubbling and hot. Let rest for 10 minutes before serving. Store any leftovers in an airtight container in the refrigerator for up to 5 days or in the freezer, tightly wrapped to avoid freezer burn, for up to 3 months.

Nutritional Information | Calories: 365 | Total Carbs: 5.1 g | Dietary Fiber: 0.8 g | Protein: 31 g | Fat: 21.7 g | Saturated Fat: 11.8 g

Tips

You can also use store-bought egg white wraps for this lasagna. And while you should try to cover most of the bottom of the pan, it's okay to have a few gaps. Once the lasagna is baked, it all holds together nicely.

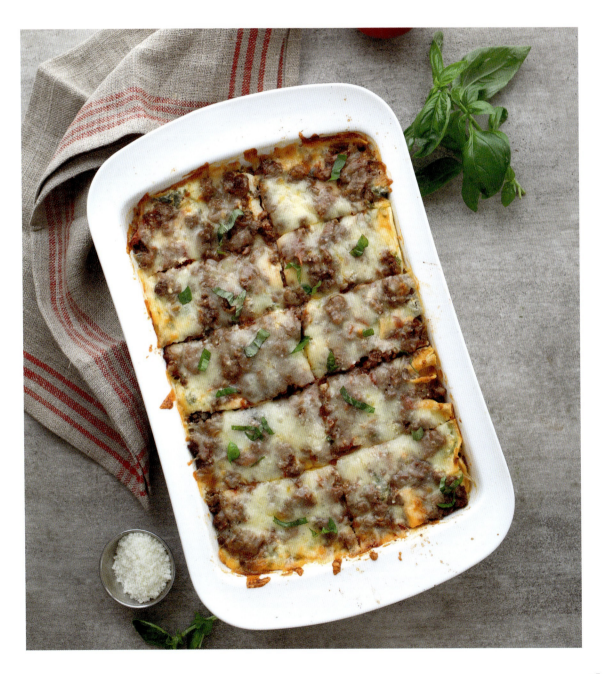

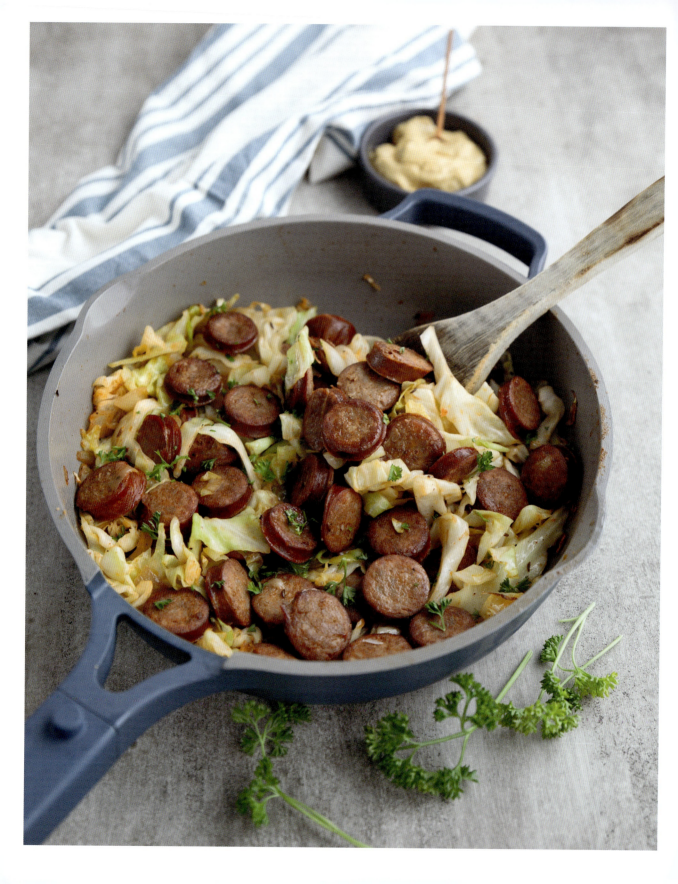

Cabbage and Smoked Sausage Skillet

Using smoked sausage is a tasty way to add flavor to any meal, and this skillet dinner is no exception. It's so quick and easy, perfect for busy weeknights.

Yield: 4 servings

Prep Time: 10 minutes

Cook Time: 14 minutes

Total Time: 24 minutes

DAIRY-FREE, EGG-FREE, NUT-FREE

2 tablespoons (28 ml) olive oil, divided

1¼ pounds (570 g) fully cooked smoked sausage, cut into ½-inch (1 cm) rounds

½ cup (80 g) chopped onion

1 teaspoon caraway seeds

½ teaspoon smoked paprika

¼ teaspoon red pepper flakes

12 ounces (340 g) cabbage, shredded

Quick protein boost:

Add some cooked shrimp or chicken when you return the sausage to the pan for a higher protein count.

1. In a large skillet over medium heat, heat 1 tablespoon (15 ml) of the oil until it shimmers. Add the sausage and sauté until nicely browned, about 4 minutes. Transfer to a plate.

2. Add the remaining 1 tablespoon (15 ml) oil to the pan along with the onion and sauté until it becomes translucent, about 2 minutes. Add the caraway seeds, paprika, and red pepper flakes and sauté for another minute.

3. Stir in the cabbage and cook until tender, about 6 minutes. Return the sausage to the pan, toss to combine, and heat through for a couple minutes before serving.

4. Store any leftovers in an airtight container in the refrigerator for up to 5 days.

Tips

- Use any kind of cooked, smoked sausage. Oftentimes it's made with beef or a mix of pork and beef; you can also use chicken or turkey sausage. Just be sure to check the labels because some are made with sugar or even high fructose corn syrup (gasp!).

- I use Teton Waters Ranch Polish Sausage and that is how the nutritional info is calculated. Keep in mind that turkey or chicken sausage will likely have even more protein and less fat.

Nutritional Information | Calories: 407 | Total Carbs: 8.9 g | Dietary Fiber: 2.8 g | Protein: 22 g | Fat: 33.1 g | Saturated Fat: 6 g

Greek Lamb Chops

Growing up in Canada, we ate the classic lamb chops with mint sauce. However, lamb lends itself well to a variety of flavors and cuisines, particularly Mediterranean and Middle Eastern. This bright lemon and garlic marinade really complements the rich meat. I love to pair these with roasted cauliflower or grilled zucchini.

Yield: 6 servings (4 ounces per serving)

Prep Time: 40 minutes (includes 30 minutes to marinate)

Cook Time: 15 minutes

Total Time: 55 minutes

DAIRY-FREE, EGG-FREE, NUT-FREE

¼ cup (60 ml) olive oil

2 teaspoons grated lemon zest

¼ cup (60 ml) freshly squeezed lemon juice

4 garlic cloves, minced

2 teaspoons chopped fresh rosemary leaves

1½ teaspoons dried marjoram

1 teaspoon dried parsley

¾ teaspoon salt

½ teaspoon ground black pepper

1½ pounds (680 g) lamb loin chops (1 inch, or 2.5 cm, thick)

1. In a large bowl, whisk the oil, lemon zest, lemon juice, garlic, rosemary, marjoram, parsley, salt, and pepper to combine. Place the lamb chops in the marinade and toss to coat. Let sit at room temperature for 30 minutes to marinate.

2. Preheat the oven to 350°F (180°C or gas mark 4).

3. Place a large ovenproof skillet over medium-high heat. Remove the chops from the marinade and put them in the skillet. Discard the used marinade. Pan-sear for about 3 minutes per side until nicely browned.

4. Place the skillet in the oven and bake for 5 to 7 minutes, depending on the chops' thickness. They should reach 130°F (54°C) on an instant-read thermometer. Transfer to a plate, tent with aluminum foil, and let rest for 5 minutes.

5. Store any leftovers in an airtight container in the refrigerator for up to 5 days.

Tips

Avoid lamb chops that are cut too thick because they are harder to cook evenly. I like chops that are 1 to 1¼ inches (2.5 to 3.2 cm) thick.

Nutritional Information | Calories: 352 | Total Carbs: 1.8 g | Dietary Fiber: 0.4 g | Protein: 29.4 g | Fat: 23.1 g | Saturated Fat: 8.6 g

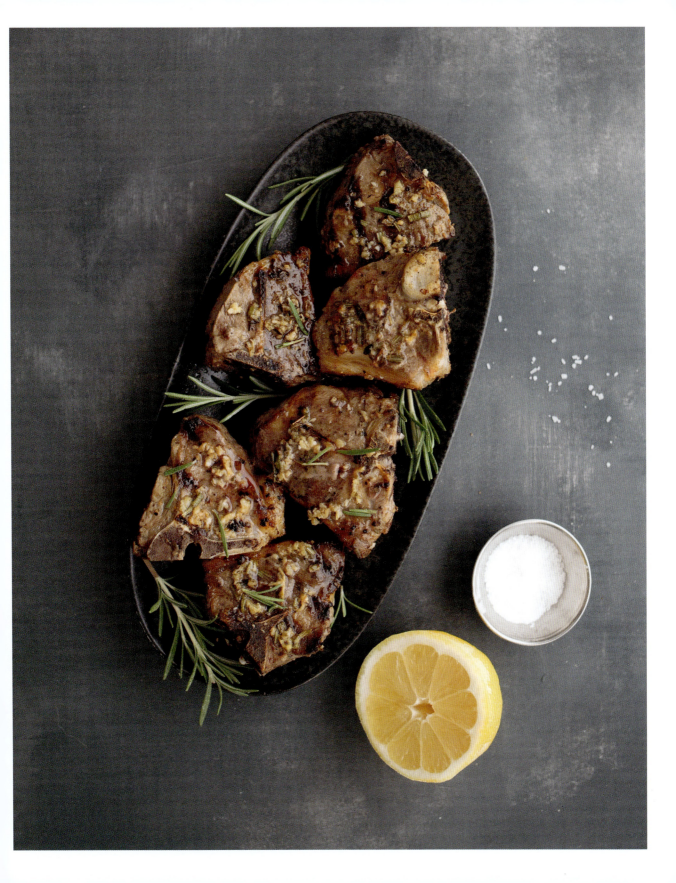

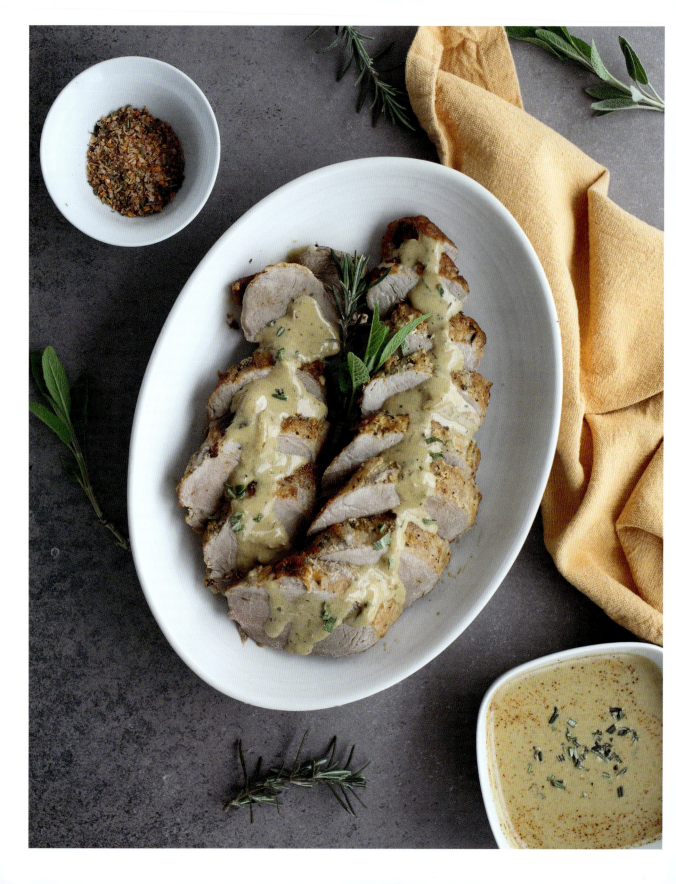

Pork Tenderloin with Dijon Cream Sauce

This creamy mustard sauce is lick-your-spoon delicious! It's also great over chicken or fish.

Yield: 6 servings

Prep Time: 5 minutes

Cook Time: 30 minutes

Total Time: 35 minutes

EGG-FREE, NUT-FREE

- 2 pounds (910 g) pork tenderloin
- Salt and ground black pepper
- 1 tablespoon (15 ml) olive oil
- 1 tablespoon (14 g) salted butter
- 1 medium-size shallot, minced
- ½ cup (120 ml) dry white wine or chicken broth
- ¼ cup (60 g) Dijon mustard
- 1 tablespoon (3 g) chopped fresh sage
- ½ cup (120 ml) heavy whipping cream

1. Preheat the oven to 425°F (220°C or gas mark 7).

2. Pat the tenderloin dry with paper towel and season it all over with salt and pepper.

3. In a large skillet over medium heat, heat the oil until it shimmers. Place the tenderloin in the skillet and brown on all sides, about 6 minutes, then transfer to a baking dish. Leave the skillet on the heat.

4. Place the baking dish in the oven and bake the pork for 18 to 25 minutes, or until it reaches 140°F (60°C) on an instant-read thermometer.

5. While the pork cooks, make the sauce. Add the butter to the hot skillet to melt, then add the shallot and sauté until tender, about 2 minutes. Pour in the wine, bring to a simmer, and cook until reduced by half, about 2 minutes. Reduce the heat to medium-low. Whisk in the mustard and sage, then whisk in the cream and cook until thickened to your liking, 2 to 3 minutes more.

6. Slice the pork into ½-inch (1 cm) slices and serve with the sauce drizzled on top.

7. Store any leftovers in an airtight container in the refrigerator for up to 5 days.

Tips

Pork tenderloin is easy to cook, but it's also easy to overcook. Check on it frequently when it's in the oven. I always recommend an instant-read thermometer when cooking recipes like this to identify the right temperature for safely cooked pork without drying it out.

Nutritional Information | Calories: 311 | Total Carbs: 2.5 g | Dietary Fiber: 0.5 g | Protein: 33.4 g | Fat: 16.1 g | Saturated Fat: 8 g

Pork Chops with Raspberry Pan Sauce

Remember how pork chops used to be served with applesauce? Turns out they go nicely with raspberries too. This raspberry sauce has the perfect tart-sweet flavor to offset the rich pork.

Yield: 4 servings

Prep Time: 10 minutes

Cook Time: 20 minutes

Total Time: 30 minutes

DAIRY-FREE, EGG-FREE, NUT-FREE

- 4 bone-in pork chops (about 1 inch, or 2.5 cm, thick)
- Salt and ground black pepper
- 2 tablespoons (28 ml) avocado oil, divided
- 1 medium-size shallot, minced
- 1 cup (125 g) raspberries, fresh or frozen, crushed
- ½ cup (120 ml) chicken broth
- 2 teaspoons balsamic vinegar

1. Pat the pork chops dry with paper towel and season them all over with salt and pepper.

2. In a large skillet over medium-high heat, heat 1 tablespoon (15 ml) of the oil until it shimmers. Add the pork chops and let sear on the first side for 4 minutes. Reduce the heat to medium and cook the chops on the second side for 7 to 10 minutes, or until the internal temperature reaches 135°F (57°C) on an instant-read thermometer. Transfer to a plate and tent with aluminum foil.

3. Add the remaining 1 tablespoon (15 ml) oil to the pan along with the shallot and sauté until it becomes tender, about 2 minutes. Add the crushed berries and the broth and bring to a simmer. Cook for 3 to 4 minutes until the pan sauce begins to thicken.

4. Remove from the heat and stir in the vinegar. Spoon the sauce over the pork chops to serve.

5. Store any leftovers in an airtight container in the refrigerator for up to 5 days.

Tips

Pork chops don't come in standard sizes, and some are absolutely ginormous. Choose medium-size chops (about 6 ounces, or 170 g) with the fat trimmed to ¼ inch (6 mm). Don't get them too thick or they become harder to cook through properly. One to 1½ inches (2.5 to 3.8 cm) is a good thickness for pan-searing.

Nutritional Information | Calories: 463 | Total Carbs: 4.7 g | Dietary Fiber: 2.1 g | Protein: 48.4 g | Fat: 28.6 g | Saturated Fat: 9.4 g

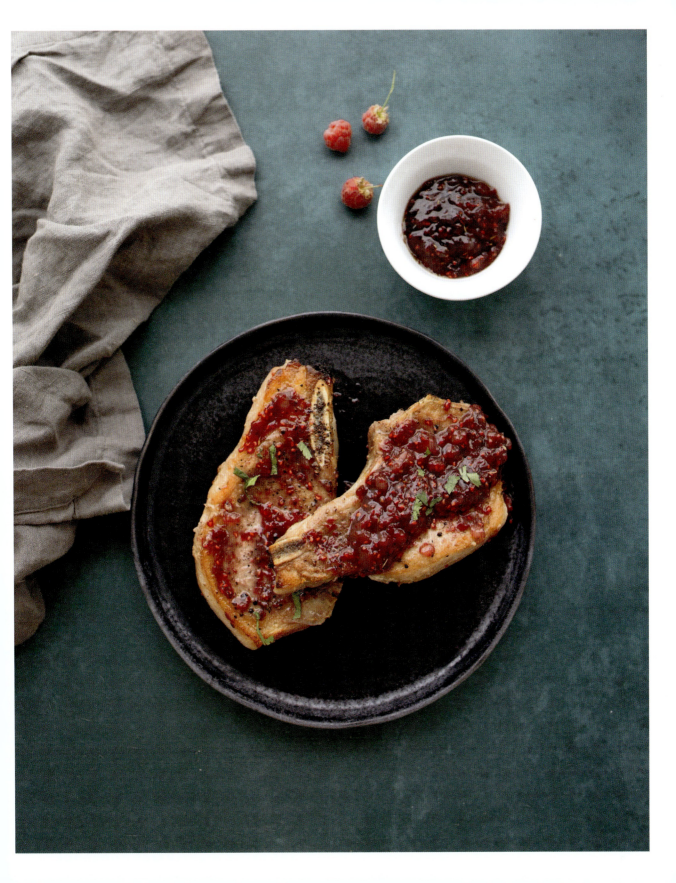

Easy Pork Stir-Fry

Sliced pork tenderloin is the perfect cut for an easy and flavorful stir-fry because it cooks quickly but remains tender.

Yield: 4 servings

Prep Time: 15 minutes

Cook Time: 15 minutes

Total Time: 30 minutes

DAIRY-FREE, EGG-FREE, NUT-FREE

FOR SAUCE:

3 tablespoons (45 ml) tamari or soy sauce

1 tablespoon (15 ml) rice vinegar

1 tablespoon (15 ml) toasted sesame oil

2 garlic cloves, minced

½ teaspoon ground ginger

¼ teaspoon red pepper flakes (optional)

FOR STIR-FRY:

1½ pounds (680 g) pork tenderloin

2 tablespoons (28 ml) avocado oil, divided

½ teaspoon salt

½ teaspoon ground black pepper

4 cups (280 g) shredded cabbage

1 medium-size red bell pepper, thinly sliced

1. To make the sauce: In a small bowl, whisk the tamari, vinegar, sesame oil, garlic, ginger, and red pepper flakes (if using) to blend.

2. To make the stir-fry: Cut the tenderloin into ½-inch (1 cm)-thick slices, then cut each slice into ½-inch (1 cm) strips.

3. In a large skillet or wok over medium-high heat, heat 1 tablespoon (15 ml) of the avocado oil. Add the tenderloin strips and season with the salt and black pepper. Stir-fry until the pork is no longer pink, 7 to 8 minutes. Transfer to a bowl.

4. Add the remaining 1 tablespoon (15 ml) avocado oil to the pan along with the cabbage and red bell pepper and sauté until the cabbage is tender, about 5 minutes.

5. Return the pork to the skillet and drizzle with the sauce. Toss to combine and cook another minute to warm through.

6. Store any leftovers in an airtight container in the refrigerator for up to 5 days.

Tips

This healthy stir-fry is great with boneless chicken thighs as well.

Nutritional Information | Calories: 305 | Total Carbs: 8 g | Dietary Fiber: 2.8 g | Protein: 39 g | Fat: 15.9 g | Saturated Fat: 3.7 g

Mediterranean Baked Cod

Cod is a very lean fish with a mild flavor, so it goes well with almost anything. Baked with tomatoes, olives, feta, and herbs, the cod becomes delightfully flaky and toothsome.

Yield: 4 servings

Prep Time: 10 minutes

Cook Time: 13 minutes

Total Time: 23 minutes

EGG-FREE, NUT-FREE

- 4 cod fillets (about 6 ounces, or 170 g, each)
- 3 tablespoons (45 ml) olive oil
- 2 tablespoons (8 g) chopped fresh parsley
- 4 garlic cloves, minced
- 2 teaspoons Dijon mustard
- 2 teaspoons grated lemon zest
- ½ teaspoon dried oregano
- ½ teaspoon paprika
- ½ teaspoon salt
- ½ teaspoon ground black pepper
- 1 cup (150 g) cherry tomatoes, halved
- ⅓ cup (50 g) crumbled feta cheese
- ⅓ cup (43 g) sliced green or black olives
- ¼ cup (29 g) sliced red onion

1. Preheat the oven to 425°F (220°C or gas mark 7) and lightly grease a glass or ceramic baking dish.

2. Arrange the cod in a single layer in the prepared dish.

3. In a small bowl, whisk the oil, parsley, garlic, mustard, lemon zest, oregano, paprika, salt, and pepper. Spread the mixture over the fillets.

4. Arrange the tomatoes, feta, olives, and onion around the fish in the baking dish.

5. Bake for 8 to 12 minutes, depending on the thickness of the fillets. For 1½-inch (3.5 cm) fillets, 9 minutes is about right. The fish should flake easily with a fork when done.

6. Turn on the broiler and cook for 30 to 60 seconds to lightly brown the tops.

7. Store any leftovers in an airtight container in the refrigerator for up to 5 days.

Tips

Choose cod fillets that are at least 1 inch (2.5 cm) thick for the best results. Thin fillets cook too quickly and the tomatoes won't have time to get soft and juicy. Halibut is another great choice for this oven-baked recipe.

Nutritional Information | Calories: 271 | Total Carbs: 5.8 g | Dietary Fiber: 1.4 g | Protein: 28.7 g | Fat: 14.2 g | Saturated Fat: 3.6 g

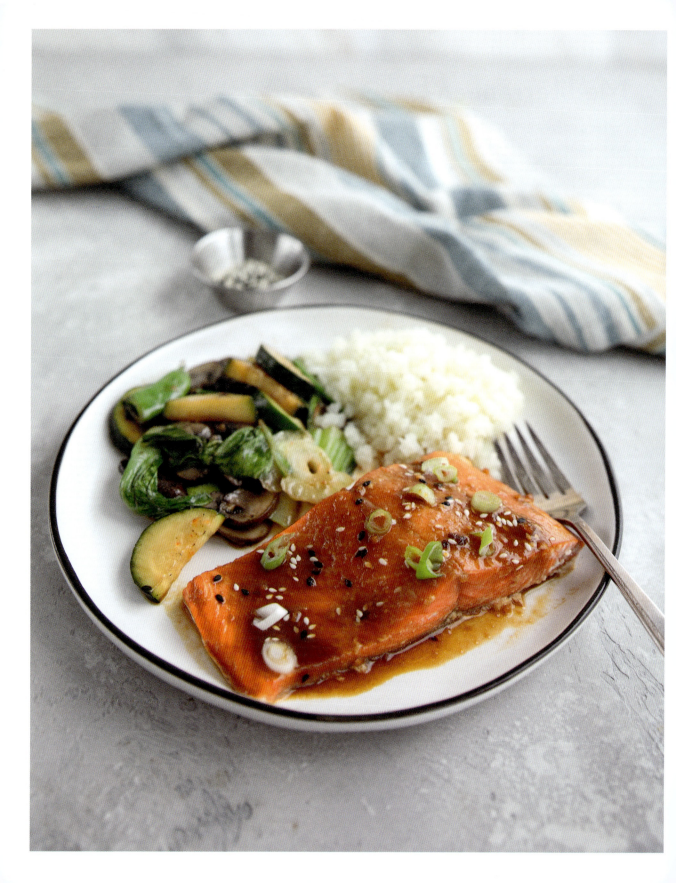

Teriyaki Salmon

Flavorful doesn't even begin to describe this baked salmon recipe. The tender, juicy fish pairs delightfully with the umami flavors of soy and sesame. Serve with some sautéed vegetables and a little cauliflower rice for a well-rounded meal.

Yield: 4 servings

Prep Time: 10 minutes

Cook Time: 20 minutes

Total Time: 30 minutes

DAIRY-FREE, EGG-FREE, NUT-FREE

¼ cup (60 ml) tamari or soy sauce

2 tablespoons (28 ml) rice vinegar

2 tablespoons (24 g) allulose granular sweetener

1 tablespoon (15 ml) sesame oil

2 garlic cloves, minced

1 teaspoon minced peeled fresh ginger

¼ teaspoon red pepper flakes

¼ teaspoon glucomannan or xanthan gum

1¼ pounds (570 g) salmon fillet, cut into 4 equal portions

Sesame seeds, for garnish

Sliced scallion, for garnish

1. In a small saucepan over medium-low heat, combine the soy sauce, vinegar, sweetener, sesame oil, garlic, ginger, and red pepper flakes. Bring to a simmer and cook for 3 to 5 minutes until slightly thickened. Remove from the heat and sprinkle the surface with glucomannan, then whisk briskly to combine. Set aside for a few minutes to cool and thicken.

2. Preheat the oven to 425°F (220°C or gas mark 7) and lightly grease a large glass or ceramic baking dish.

3. Arrange the salmon in a single layer in the prepared dish and pour about half of the sauce over the fillets, brushing to coat the top of each.

4. Bake for 9 to 12 minutes, depending on the thickness of the fish. The salmon should be opaque and flake easily with a fork when done.

5. Brush the tops with the remaining sauce and sprinkle with sesame seeds and scallion to serve.

6. Store any leftovers in an airtight container in the refrigerator for up to 5 days.

Tips

The best low-carb sweetener for a sauce like this is allulose because it becomes more syrupy, like real teriyaki, and it doesn't recrystallize. That said, use any granular sweetener in this recipe.

Nutritional Information | Calories: 309 | Total Carbs: 1.7 g | Dietary Fiber: 0.3 g | Protein: 30.2 g | Fat: 14 g | Saturated Fat: 3.2 g

Shrimp Fried Cauliflower Rice

Nothing beats this flavorful shrimp fried "rice" recipe for a quick and easy weeknight meal. And it won't weigh you down like the takeout version!

Yield: 4 servings

Prep Time: 12 minutes

Cook Time: 12 minutes

Total Time: 24 minutes

DAIRY-FREE, NUT-FREE

- 2 tablespoons (28 ml) sesame or avocado oil
- 1 pound (455 g) medium-size peeled shrimp, tails removed
- ¾ teaspoon salt
- ½ teaspoon ground black pepper
- ¼ teaspoon red pepper flakes
- ½ medium-size orange or red bell pepper, finely chopped
- 2 scallions, white and green parts, thinly sliced (save some green parts for garnish)
- 2 garlic cloves, minced
- ½ teaspoon minced peeled fresh ginger
- 3 large eggs, beaten
- 16 ounces (455 g) frozen cauliflower rice, thawed
- 2 tablespoons (28 ml) tamari or soy sauce
- 1 tablespoon (15 ml) toasted sesame oil

1. In a large skillet over medium-high heat, heat 1 tablespoon (15 ml) of the sesame oil until it shimmers. Add the shrimp in a single layer and season with the salt, black pepper, and red pepper flakes. Cook for 1 minute, flip, and cook for another minute until the shrimp are bright pink. Transfer to a bowl.

2. Add the remaining 1 tablespoon (15 ml) sesame oil to the pan along with the bell pepper, scallions, garlic, and ginger and sauté for 2 minutes.

3. Push the veggies to one side of the pan and add the eggs to the open part of the skillet. Use a spatula to scramble the eggs quickly.

4. Add the cauliflower rice to the pan and stir-fry quickly to combine. Cook for 3 minutes, then return the shrimp to the skillet and add the tamari and toasted sesame oil. Sauté for another minute to warm through. Garnish with the reserved scallion greens.

5. Store any leftovers in an airtight container in the refrigerator for up to 5 days.

Tips

Shrimp is a great addition to almost any meal when you need to add a little protein. About 3½ ounces (100 g) of shrimp has only 99 calories, 0.2 grams of carbs, and a whopping 24 grams of protein. It's also quick and easy to cook!

Nutritional Information | Calories: 252 | Total Carbs: 8 g | Dietary Fiber: 3.2 g | Protein: 30.8 g | Fat: 14.1 g | Saturated Fat: 2.9 g

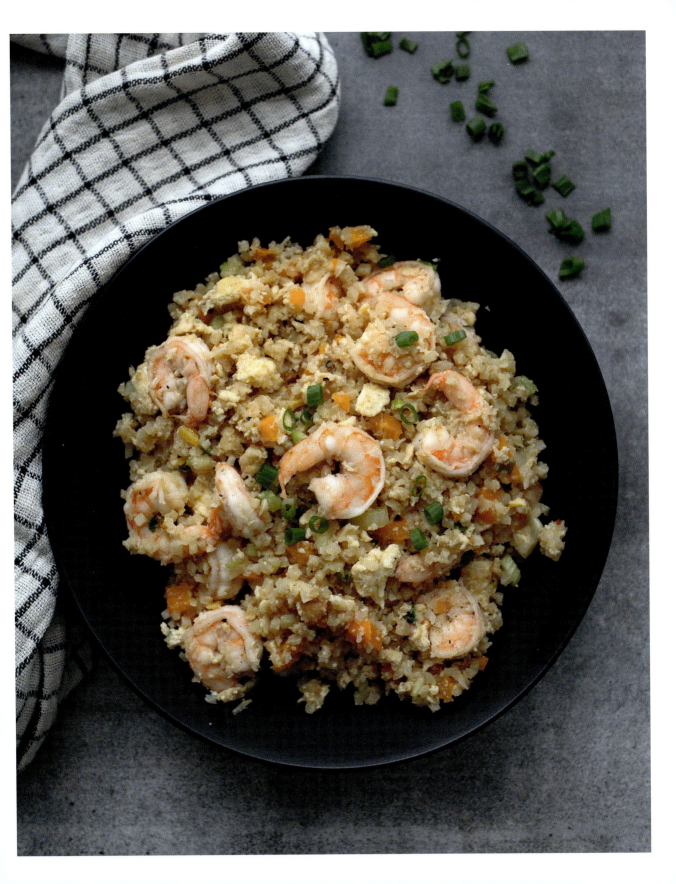

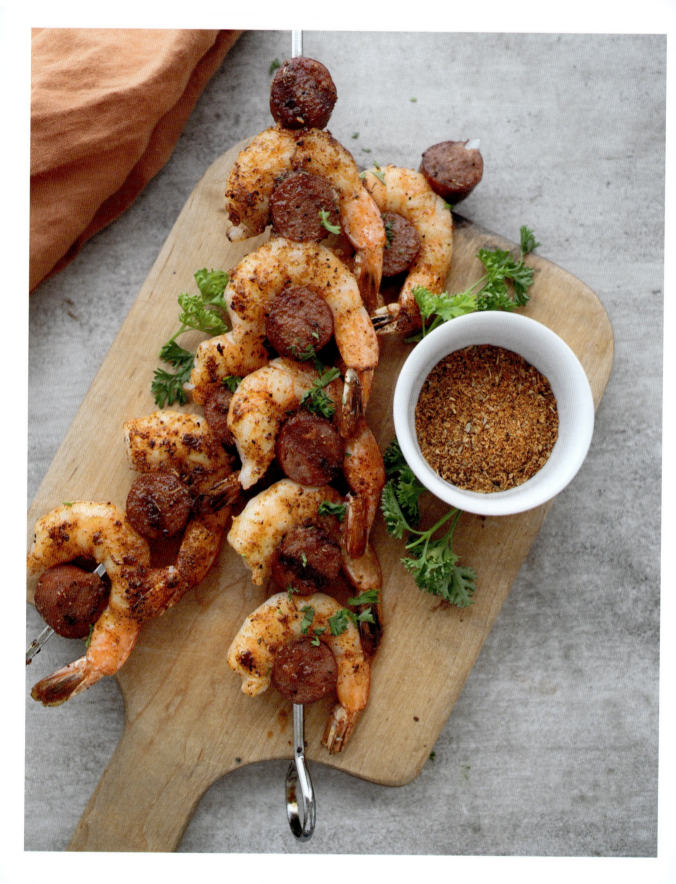

Shrimp and Sausage Skewers

Ready in 20 minutes, this Cajun-style meal is the ultimate easy summer dinner. And it takes only 4 ingredients!

Yield: 6 servings

Prep Time: 10 minutes

Cook Time: 10 minutes

Total Time: 20 minutes

EGG-FREE, NUT-FREE

4 tablespoons (55 g) salted butter, melted

1 tablespoon (12 g) Cajun seasoning

12 ounces (340 g) fully cooked smoked sausage

1½ pounds (680 g) raw large shrimp, peeled and deveined

Salt and ground black pepper

1. If using bamboo skewers, soak 6 skewers in water for 1 hour before cooking so they don't burn on the grill.

2. Preheat a grill to medium-high heat.

3. In a small bowl, whisk the melted butter and Cajun seasoning to blend.

4. Cut each sausage into 9 slices so you have 36 pieces. Thread 1 slice on each skewer, cut-side facing out. Thread a shrimp onto a skewer so it curls around the sausage. Repeat with 4 more sausage slices and 4 more shrimp per skewer. Cap each skewer with a final slice of sausage. Each skewer should have 6 slices of sausage and 5 shrimp. Brush both sides of each skewer with the butter mixture.

5. Place the skewers on the grill over direct heat and cook until the shrimp are pink and cooked through, 3 to 5 minutes per side. Alternatively, you can cook the skewers under a preheated broiler for 3 to 5 minutes per side. Season to taste with salt and pepper.

6. Store any leftovers in an airtight container in the refrigerator for up to 5 days.

Tips

You need fully cooked sausage for this recipe because shrimp cook so quickly on the grill. Smoked sausage, like kielbasa or andouille, is my preference.

Nutritional Information | Calories: 273 | Total Carbs: 1.5 g | Dietary Fiber: 0 g | Protein: 29.1 g | Fat: 16.6 g | Saturated Fat: 5 g

Cloud Bread Protein Pizza

Who says you can't enjoy pizza on a high-protein, low-carb diet? The crust of this cloud bread pizza is almost pure protein. And up the protein even more by adding chicken or sausage to your toppings!

Yield: 4 servings

Prep Time: 20 minutes

Cook Time: 30 minutes

Total Time: 50 minutes

NUT-FREE

FOR CRUST:

4 large egg whites

½ teaspoon cream of tartar

½ teaspoon salt

2 ounces (55 g) cream cheese, softened

1 large egg, at room temperature

6 tablespoons (45 g) unflavored whey protein powder

1 teaspoon pizza seasoning

½ teaspoon garlic powder

FOR PIZZA:

⅓ cup (82 g) tomato sauce

½ cup (115 g) shredded mozzarella

2 ounces (55 g) pepperoni

2 medium-size mushrooms, thinly sliced

Sliced bell peppers, olives, pepperoncini, or other favorite pizza toppings (optional)

1. Preheat the oven to 350°F (180°C or gas mark 4) and lightly grease a large baking sheet. Line the pan with parchment paper and lightly grease the parchment.

2. To make the crust: In a large bowl, using a handheld electric mixer, beat the egg whites with the cream of tartar and salt on medium-high speed until they hold stiff peaks.

3. In a blender or food processor, combine the cream cheese, whole egg, protein powder, pizza seasoning, and garlic powder. Blend until smooth. Carefully fold the cream cheese mixture into the whipped egg whites until no streaks remain. Spread the mixture into a 12-inch (30 cm) circle on the prepared baking sheet, making the sides slightly higher than the center.

4. Bake for 12 to 15 minutes until firm to the touch. Remove from the oven and increase the oven temperature to 400°F (200°C or gas mark 6).

5. To assemble the pizza: Spread the crust with the tomato sauce, sprinkle with the cheese, and arrange the pepperoni, mushrooms, and any other toppings as desired on top.

6. Bake for 12 to 15 minutes until the cheese is melted and bubbling. Let cool a few minutes before slicing.

7. Store any leftovers in an airtight container in the refrigerator for up to 5 days.

Nutritional Information | Calories: 281 | Total Carbs: 5.4 g | Dietary Fiber: 0.4 g | Protein: 22.3 g | Fat: 16.7 g | Saturated Fat: 9.2 g

Tips

- You can use carton egg whites for this recipe, but they may take a bit longer to whip into stiff peaks.

- Greasing the pan before laying down the parchment helps it stay in place as you spread the crust mixture.

- Choose a tomato sauce with no added sugar, like Rao's Marinara. It should have no more than 5 grams of carbs per ½ cup (125 g).

Protein powder options

The crust works best with whey protein, as egg white protein makes it a bit rubbery. You could also try some plant-based protein powders, but they may change the flavor and appearance.

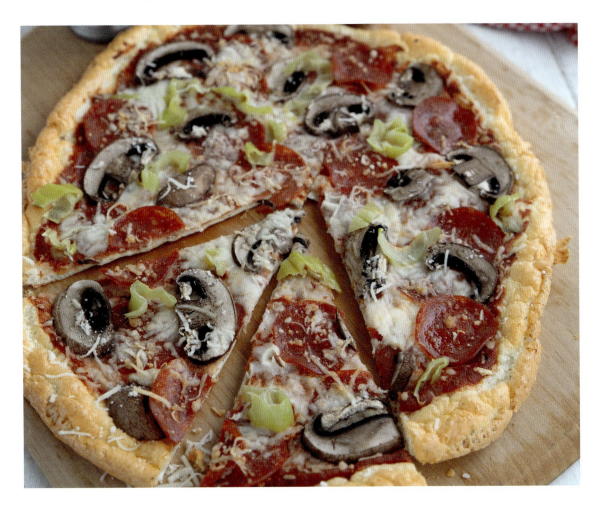

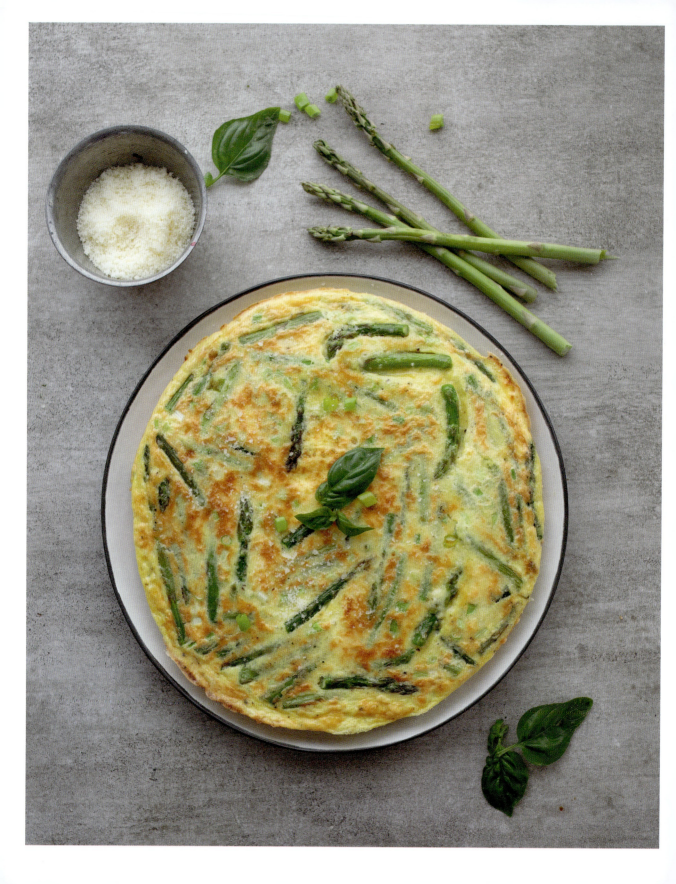

Asparagus Parmesan Frittata

Frittata is one of those simple but elegant meals that always tastes fantastic. It also makes an excellent brunch!

Yield: 4 servings

Prep Time: 10 minutes

Cook Time: 20 minutes

Total Time: 30 minutes

NUT-FREE, VEGETARIAN

- 1 tablespoon (14 g) salted butter
- 1 tablespoon (15 ml) olive oil
- 1 pound (455 g) asparagus, trimmed and cut into 2-inch (5 cm) pieces
- 2 garlic cloves, minced
- 10 large eggs
- ⅔ cup (240 g) high-protein yogurt
- ½ cup (50 g) grated parmesan cheese, divided
- 2 scallions, white and green parts, sliced
- ½ teaspoon salt
- ½ teaspoon ground black pepper

1. In a 10-inch (25 cm) ovenproof skillet set over medium heat, melt the butter with the oil until hot. Add the asparagus and sauté until tender and bright green, about 4 minutes. Add the garlic and cook for another minute until fragrant. Remove from the heat.

2. In a large bowl, whisk the eggs and yogurt until well combined. Stir in 6 tablespoons (30 g) of the parmesan, the scallions, salt, and pepper. Pour the egg mixture over the asparagus in the pan. Shake the skillet gently to distribute the ingredients evenly.

3. Place the skillet over medium-low heat and cook for 8 to 10 minutes until the edges are set but the center is still loose.

4. Adjust an oven rack to the second-highest position and preheat the broiler to high.

5. Sprinkle the remaining 2 tablespoons (10 g) parmesan over the frittata.

6. Broil the frittata until puffed and golden brown, 2 to 5 minutes, watching carefully to make sure it doesn't burn.

7. Store any leftovers in an airtight container in the refrigerator for up to 5 days.

Tips

- Not an asparagus fan? Swap it for another low-carb vegetable, like broccoli. You can also swap the yogurt for blended cottage cheese.

- Parmesan cheese has a surprising amount of protein for something we often sprinkle on as an afterthought. One ounce (28 g) of parmesan contains 10 grams of protein.

Nutritional Information | Calories: 334 | Total Carbs: 7.5 g | Dietary Fiber: 2.6 g | Protein: 26.4 g | Fat: 20.9 g | Saturated Fat: 8.6 g

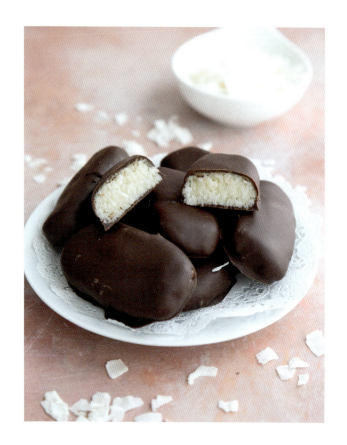

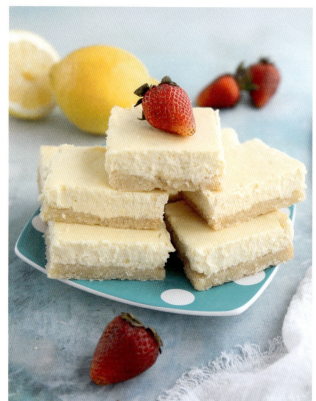

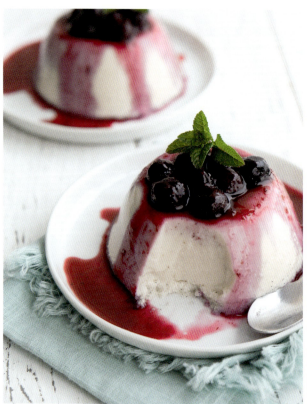

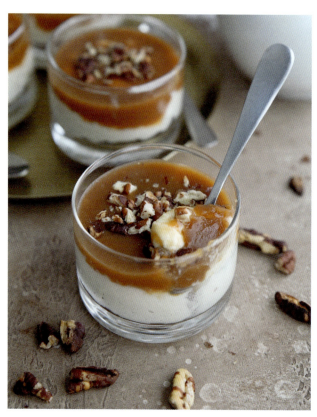

CHAPTER 9

DESSERTS

If the majority of your protein comes from your meals, is it even necessary to consume high-protein desserts? Perhaps not, but it sure is fun! If you know my work, you know I love to bake. And I love the challenge of creating healthier desserts that look and taste like the high-carb, high-sugar versions. Why not make desserts that pack in some extra protein while I'm at it? Enjoying a Chocolate Chip Cookie (page 194) that has 11 grams of protein and doesn't spike my blood sugar brings me great joy.

People are often surprised to learn that I eat a little dessert every day—emphasis on a *little*. It's important to exercise moderation and remember that desserts are special treats, even if they are sugar free. If sweet foods trigger you and cause you to crave more or overeat, you may want to skip the recipes in this chapter.

For many people, eating a little sweet at the end of the day helps keep them from feeling deprived. If you love creamy desserts, try the Lemon Cheesecake Bars (page 202) or the Raspberry Ricotta Custard (page 204). Cool off on a hot day with a refreshing Strawberry Lemonade Ice Pops (page 212). And the Frosted Chocolate Cake (page 198) is perfect for special occasions.

Chocolate Chip Cookies

What's better than a tender chocolate chip cookie? One that packs an added protein punch, of course! Sometimes, I smear these with a little peanut butter or the Chocolate Hazelnut Spread on page 121.

Yield: 24 cookies (2 cookies per serving)

Prep Time: 15 minutes

Cook Time: 12 minutes

Total Time: 27 minutes

DAIRY-FREE OPTION, VEGETARIAN OPTION

1 cup (112 g) almond flour

⅔ cup (80 g) whey protein powder

1 tablespoon (7 g) grass-fed gelatin (optional)

½ teaspoon baking soda

¼ teaspoon salt

½ cup (130 g) almond butter

4 tablespoons (55 g) unsalted butter or coconut oil (dairy-free option), at room temperature

½ cup (96 g) brown sugar substitute

1 large egg

1 teaspoon vanilla extract

½ cup (120 g) sugar-free chocolate chips, divided

Protein powder options

Experiment with other protein powders, but keep in mind that collagen and bone broth protein may not provide a full amino acid profile.

1. Preheat the oven to 325°F (170°C or gas mark 3) and line 2 baking sheets with silicone mats or parchment paper.

2. In a medium bowl, whisk the almond flour, protein powder, gelatin (if using), baking soda, and salt to combine.

3. In a large bowl, using a handheld electric mixer, beat together the almond butter and butter on medium speed until well combined, then beat in the brown sugar substitute. Add the egg and vanilla and beat until smooth. Add the dry ingredients and beat until the dough comes together.

4. Stir in about one-third of the chocolate chips by hand. Form the dough into 24 balls about 1 inch (2.5 cm) in diameter and place them on the prepared baking sheets 2 inches (5 cm) apart. Press the cookies down lightly with the palm of your hand so they're about ¾ inch (2 cm) thick. Press the remaining chocolate chips into the tops of the cookies.

5. Bake for 10 to 12 minutes until puffed and just turning brown around the edges. The tops will still be very soft. Let cool completely on the pan.

6. Store the cookies in an airtight container on the counter for up to 4 days or in the refrigerator for up to 1 week.

Nutritional Information | Calories: 218 | Total Carbs: 7.8 g | Dietary Fiber: 4.7 g | Protein: 11 g | Fat: 17 g | Saturated Fat: 5.5 g

Tips

- The grass-fed gelatin helps give the cookies a chewier consistency. Omit it, if you prefer.

- It's better to err on the side of undercooking these cookies, as baked goods with protein powder can dry out if overbaked. Leave them on the pan until they are completely cool, or they will be impossible to pick up!

- I think these cookies taste best with a brown sugar substitute, but any sweetener should work. Don't pack the sweetener because you will end up with too much.

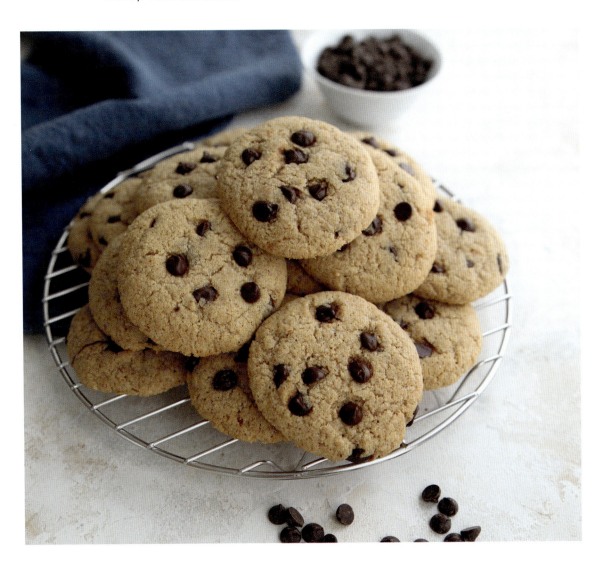

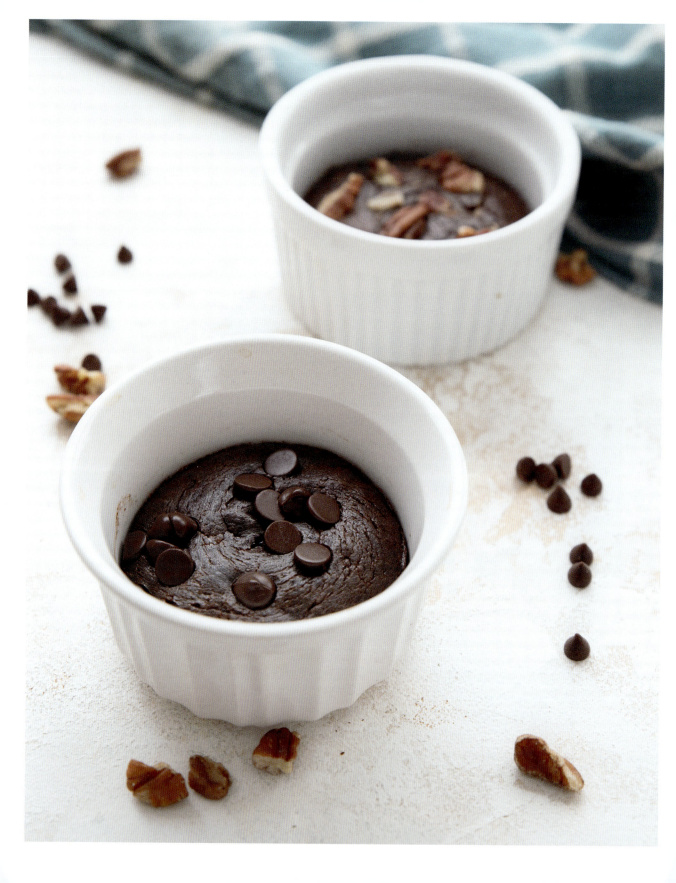

Deep-Dish Brownies

These warm, gooey brownies are meant to be eaten right out of the dish. You can also make them in a small countertop oven or an air fryer. Add a little low-carb ice cream for a serious indulgence! And because peanuts, sunflower seeds, and pumpkin seeds all contain tryptophan, they have a complete amino acid profile.

Yield: 4 servings

Prep Time: 10 minutes

Cook Time: 14 minutes

Total Time: 24 minutes

DAIRY-FREE, NUT-FREE OPTION

- ¼ cup (65 g) creamy natural peanut butter
- 1 tablespoon (15 ml) avocado oil
- 3 tablespoons (24 g) sweetener (granular or powdered)
- ½ teaspoon vanilla extract
- 2 tablespoons (28 ml) whisked egg
- 3½ tablespoons (25 g) collagen protein powder
- 1 tablespoon (5 g) cocoa powder
- ¼ teaspoon baking powder
- Pinch salt
- 2 to 4 tablespoons (28 to 60 ml) water or brewed coffee
- 2 tablespoons (15 g) sugar-free chocolate chips or chopped nuts (optional)

1. Preheat the oven to 325°F (170°C or gas mark 3) and lightly grease four ½-cup (120 ml) ramekins.

2. In a medium microwave-safe bowl, melt the peanut butter with the oil on high power in 30-second increments, stirring until smooth. Stir in the sweetener and vanilla, then stir in the egg. The mixture may become very thick at this point.

3. All at once, add the collagen, cocoa powder, baking powder, and salt and work the ingredients in until well combined. Stir in the water, 1 tablespoon (15 ml) at a time, until you have a thick but pourable batter. Divide the batter among the prepared ramekins and top with chocolate chips or nuts (if using).

4. Bake for 10 to 14 minutes, depending on how gooey you like brownies. Let cool for 5 minutes before serving.

Tips

- For brownies that are almost molten, bake for 9 to 10 minutes. For cakey brownies, bake for 12 to 14 minutes.

- If you are allergic to peanut butter, try sunflower seed butter or pumpkin seed butter.

Protein powder options

These brownies work best with collagen or bone broth protein for a tender consistency.

Nutritional Information | Calories: 201 | Total Carbs: 7.1 g | Dietary Fiber: 3.2 g | Protein: 16 g | Fat: 14.1 g | Saturated Fat: 3.7 g

Frosted Chocolate Cake

Sometimes you just need a delicious slice of rich chocolate cake with a decadent chocolate frosting. And this delicious high-protein cake meets the moment.

Yield: 10 slices (1 slice per serving)

Prep Time: 55 minutes (includes 30 minutes to chill)

Cook Time: 22 minutes

Total Time: 1 hour 17 minutes

VEGETARIAN

FOR CAKE:

⅔ cup (160 g) high-protein yogurt

3 large eggs

¼ cup (60 ml) avocado oil

1 teaspoon vanilla extract

1 cup (112 g) almond flour

½ cup (48 g) chocolate protein powder

⅓ cup (64 g) granular sweetener

¼ cup (20 g) cocoa powder

1 teaspoon baking powder

¼ teaspoon salt

Water or cold brewed coffee, as needed

FOR FROSTING:

4 ounces (115 g) cream cheese, softened

¾ cup (175 ml) heavy whipping cream, chilled

⅓ cup (32 g) chocolate protein powder

1. Preheat the oven to 325°F (170°C or gas mark 3) and grease a 9-inch (23 cm) round metal baking pan. Line the bottom with parchment paper and grease the parchment.

2. To make the cake: In a large bowl, whisk the yogurt, eggs, oil, and vanilla until smooth. Add the almond flour, protein powder, granular sweetener, cocoa powder, baking powder, and salt and whisk until well combined. If the batter is very thick, stir in water, 1 tablespoon (15 ml) at a time, until it is a thick but pourable consistency. Spread the batter evenly in the prepared pan.

3. Bake for 18 to 22 minutes until the top is just barely set. Do not overbake the cake because it will dry out. Let cool for 30 minutes in the pan, then run a sharp knife around the edges to loosen. Flip the cake onto a wire rack to finish cooling.

4. To make the frosting: In a large bowl, using a handheld electric mixer, beat the cream cheese on medium speed until very smooth and creamy. Turn the mixer to low speed and slowly drizzle in the cream. Once combined, add the protein powder, powdered sweetener, and cocoa powder and return the mixer to medium speed. Beat until the frosting holds stiff peaks. Add the milk, 1 tablespoon (15 ml) at a time, to thin the frosting to a nice spreadable consistency.

Nutritional Information | Calories: 263 | Total Carbs: 6.8 g | Dietary Fiber: 2.3 g | Protein: 14.4 g | Fat: 23.4 g | Saturated Fat: 9 g

¼ cup (32 g) powdered sweetener

2 tablespoons (10 g) cocoa powder

1 to 2 tablespoons (15 to 28 ml) unsweetened almond milk

5. To assemble the cake: Place the cake on a cake plate and spread the frosting over the top. Refrigerate for 30 minutes to firm up a bit before slicing. Store the cake, covered, in the refrigerator for up to 5 days.

Tips

- Dutch-process cocoa works best in low-carb cakes like this because it has a much deeper chocolate flavor and it mixes better into the other ingredients.

- Cream cheese in the frosting provides structure without using copious amounts of powdered sweetener.

Protein powder options

You can use whey, egg white, or vegan protein powders, but collagen and bone broth will make this cake very gummy and overly moist. If you don't have chocolate protein, use plain or vanilla and add an additional tablespoon (5 g) of cocoa powder to both the cake and the frosting. You may want to add some additional sweetener too.

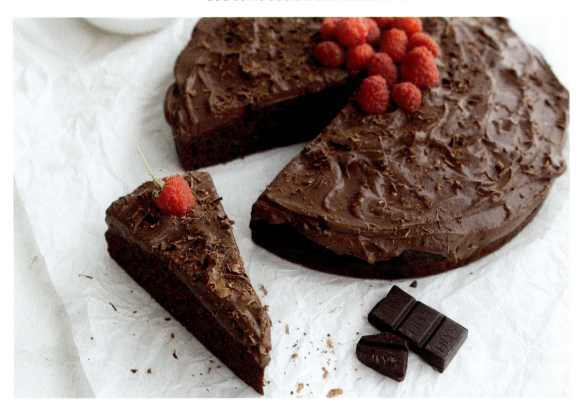

No-Bake Cookie Dough Bars

Remember sneaking bits of cookie dough from the bowl when you were a kid? Or maybe when you were an adult too? Well now you have full permission to enjoy, guilt-free!

Yield: 16 bars (1 bar per serving)

Prep Time: 1 hour 20 minutes (includes 1 hour to chill)

Total Time: 1 hour 20 minutes

DAIRY-FREE, EGG-FREE OPTION

FOR BARS:

1⅔ cups (186 g) almond flour

⅔ cup (75 g) egg white protein powder or plant-based protein powder (egg-free option)

½ cup (64 g) powdered sweetener

⅓ cup (37 g) collagen protein powder

¼ teaspoon salt

⅓ cup (80 ml) avocado oil

¼ cup (60 ml) warm water, plus more as needed

1 teaspoon vanilla extract

½ cup (120 g) sugar-free chocolate chips

FOR TOPPING:

3 ounces (85 g) sugar-free chocolate, chopped

2 teaspoons avocado oil

1. Line a 9 × 9-inch (23 × 23 cm) baking pan with parchment paper or wax paper with overhanging edges for easy removal.

2. To make the bars: In a large bowl, whisk the almond flour, egg white protein powder, powdered sweetener, collagen protein powder, and salt to blend.

3. In a small bowl, stir together the oil, warm water, and vanilla. Stir the liquid into the dry ingredients with a rubber spatula, working them together until a stiff dough forms. Stir in the chocolate chips until well distributed. If the dough seems too dry or crumbly, add more water, 1 tablespoon (15 ml) at a time. You should be able to squeeze some dough and have it hold together. Press the dough evenly into the prepared pan and use a flat-bottomed glass to even it out. Freeze for 1 hour.

4. To make the topping: In a microwave-safe bowl, melt together the chocolate and oil on high power in 30-second increments, stirring until smooth. Spread the chocolate over the chilled bars and let set for a few minutes. Use the parchment to lift the dough from the pan, then cut into 16 bars.

5. Store the bars in an airtight container in the refrigerator for up to 10 days.

Tips

You really need a powdered sweetener to avoid any grittiness in this no-bake recipe. You could also try stevia or monk fruit extract, but the bars may be a little on the soft side. If the dough is too soft, add 1 to 2 tablespoons (7 to 14 g) coconut flour.

Nutritional Information | Calories: 177 | Total Carbs: 7.6 g | Dietary Fiber: 4.4 g | Protein: 11.3 g | Fat: 15.5 g

Cannoli Dessert Dip

Love cannoli? This keto dessert dip is a fun way to enjoy all those flavors in a healthier fashion. Serve with fresh strawberries or small low-carb cookies for dipping. I also have a wonderful recipe for sugar-free graham crackers on my website.

Yield: 8 servings

Prep Time: 1 hour 15 minutes (includes 1 hour to drain)

Total Time: 1 hour 15 minutes

EGG-FREE, NUT-FREE, VEGETARIAN

⅔ cup (150 g) cottage cheese

6 ounces (170 g) cream cheese, softened

⅔ cup (80 g) vanilla protein powder

¼ cup (32 g) powdered sweetener, plus more for garnish (optional)

½ cup (120 ml) heavy whipping cream

⅓ cup (80 g) sugar-free chocolate chips, plus 1 tablespoon (15 g)

1. Place the cottage cheese in a fine-mesh sieve set over the sink or a bowl and let drain for 1 hour. Transfer to a food processor. Add the cream cheese and blend until smooth. Transfer the mixture to a medium-size bowl and whisk in the protein powder and sweetener.

2. In another medium-size bowl, using a handheld electric mixer, beat the cream on medium-high speed until it holds stiff peaks. Fold the whipped cream into the cottage cheese mixture until no streaks remain. Fold in ⅓ cup (80 g) of the chocolate chips. Transfer to a serving dish and sprinkle with the remaining 1 tablespoon (15 g) chocolate chips and a little additional powdered sweetener, if desired.

Tips

You need to use a sweetener that won't make the mixture gritty. I prefer a powdered bulk sweetener, but concentrated sweeteners like stevia or monk fruit work too.

Protein powder options

You should be able to use your favorite protein powder here, including whey, egg white, or plant-based protein. If you are using an unflavored protein, add 1 teaspoon vanilla extract and additional sweetener to taste.

Nutritional Information | Calories: 213 | Total Carbs: 6.2 g | Dietary Fiber: 3 g | Protein: 12.3 g | Fat: 15.2 g | Saturated Fat: 10 g

Lemon Cheesecake Bars

These cheesecake bars are a lemon lover's dream. They feature creamy lemon filling baked on a low-carb shortbread crust. And they pack a good amount of protein too! See top right of page 192 for photo.

Yield: 12 bars (1 bar per serving)

Prep Time: 3 hours 25 minutes (includes 3 hours to chill)

Cook Time: 47 minutes

Total Time: 4 hours 12 minutes

VEGETARIAN

FOR CRUST:

1¼ cups (140 g) almond flour

¼ cup (48 g) erythritol sweetener

¼ teaspoon salt

4 tablespoons (55 g) salted butter, melted

FOR FILLING:

8 ounces (225 g) cottage cheese

8 ounces (225 g) cream cheese, softened

⅔ cup (128 g) sweetener, plus more as needed

⅔ cup (80 g) whey protein powder

Grated zest of 1 lemon

1½ teaspoons lemon extract, plus more as needed

½ teaspoon vanilla extract

2 large eggs, at room temperature

1 tablespoon (7 g) coconut flour

1. Preheat the oven to 325°F (170°C or gas mark 3).

2. To make the crust: In a large bowl, whisk the almond flour, erythritol sweetener, and salt to blend. Stir in the melted butter until well combined. Press the crust mixture evenly into the bottom of an 8-inch (20 cm) square pan and bake for 12 minutes. Let cool completely.

3. Reduce the oven temperature to 300°F (150°C or gas mark 2).

4. To make the filling: In a food processor, combine the cottage cheese and cream cheese. Blend until smooth, stopping to scrape down the sides and bottom of the bowl as needed.

5. Add the sweetener, protein powder, lemon zest, lemon extract, and vanilla and blend until well combined. At this point, taste the mixture and adjust the sweetener and flavor as desired.

6. Add the eggs and blend until smooth, stopping to scrape down the sides and bottom of the bowl as needed. Add the coconut flour and pulse to incorporate. Pour the filling over the crust and spread it to the edges.

7. Bake for 30 to 35 minutes, or until the filling is just set and the center jiggles just slightly when shaken. Let cool completely, then refrigerate for 3 hours to firm up.

8. Store the bars in an airtight container in the refrigerator for up to 1 week.

Nutritional Information | Calories: 217 | Total Carbs: 4.6 g | Dietary Fiber: 1.5 g | Protein: 12.3 g | Fat: 16.4 g | Saturated Fat: 7.3 g

Pecan Pie Cheesecake Jars

Creamy no-bake cheesecake with a rich caramel pecan topping? This might be one of my favorite desserts in this cookbook. And it's a perfect high-protein treat for the holiday season. See bottom right of page 192 for photo.

Yield: 6 servings

Prep Time: 20 minutes

Cook Time: 10 minutes

Total Time: 30 minutes

EGG-FREE, VEGETARIAN

FOR TOPPING:

½ cup (55 g) chopped pecans

4 tablespoons (55 g) unsalted butter

2 tablespoons (24 g) brown sugar substitute

2 tablespoons (24 g) allulose granular or xylitol sweetener

¼ cup (60 ml) heavy whipping cream

⅛ teaspoon salt

FOR CHEESECAKE:

½ cup (113 g) cottage cheese

5 ounces (140 g) cream cheese, softened

½ teaspoon vanilla extract

½ cup (60 g) unflavored whey protein powder

⅓ cup (43 g) powdered sweetener

1. To make the topping: In a small skillet over medium heat, toast the pecans, stirring frequently, until they become fragrant, 5 to 7 minutes. Remove from the heat and continue to stir occasionally as they cool.

2. In a small saucepan over medium-low heat, combine the butter, brown sugar substitute, and allulose. Bring to a boil, stirring frequently. Cook for about 1 minute until the mixture begins to darken. Remove from the heat and whisk in the cream.

3. Return the mixture to the heat and bring to a simmer. Cook for 1 to 2 minutes until the mixture thickens slightly. Remove from the heat and stir in the salt.

4. To make the cheesecake: In a blender, blend the cottage cheese until smooth.

5. In a medium bowl, using a handheld electric mixer, beat the cream cheese on medium-high speed for about 1 minute until very smooth. Add the cottage cheese and vanilla and beat until well combined. Beat in the protein powder and powdered sweetener.

6. Spoon about 1 tablespoon (7 g) of the toasted pecans into the bottom of 6 small dessert cups. Divide the cream cheese mixture among the cups, then top with the caramel sauce and the remaining pecans. Serve immediately or refrigerate until ready to serve.

Tips

Brown sugar replacement gives the caramel sauce more flavor, while allulose helps keep it gooey. A powdered or liquid sweetener works best in the filling so it's not gritty.

Nutritional Information | Calories: 247 | Total Carbs: 3.7 g | Dietary Fiber: 0.9 g | Protein: 12.5 g | Fat: 20.1 g | Saturated Fat: 10.4 g

Raspberry Ricotta Custard

Grab a spoon and dig into this silky smooth baked custard. The fresh berries contrast delightfully with the creamy sweetness.

Yield: 4 servings

Prep Time: 15 minutes

Cook Time: 35 minutes

Total Time: 50 minutes

NUT-FREE, VEGETARIAN

1 cup (250 g) whole milk ricotta cheese

¼ cup (60 ml) heavy whipping cream

2 large eggs

1 large egg yolk

⅓ cup (40 g) unflavored whey protein powder

⅓ cup (43 g) powdered sweetener

2 teaspoons grated lemon zest

¼ teaspoon salt

¾ cup (94 g) fresh raspberries

Protein powder options

Egg white protein powder should also work in this recipe.

1. Preheat the oven to 350°F (180°C or gas mark 4) and set four ½-cup (120 ml) ramekins in a large baking dish.

2. In a blender, combine the ricotta, cream, eggs, egg yolk, protein powder, sweetener, lemon zest, and salt. Blend briefly to combine and let rest for 5 minutes to thicken.

3. Divide the mixture evenly among the ramekins, then top with the raspberries, allowing some of them to sink down into the mixture.

4. Fill the baking dish with enough hot water to reach halfway up the sides of the ramekins. Do not get any water inside the ramekins. Carefully place the whole baking dish into the oven.

5. Bake 30 to 35 minutes, or until the tops are golden brown and lightly puffed. A knife inserted in the center should come out clean but the custard should still jiggle slightly when shaken. Remove the baking dish from the oven and remove the custards from the water. Let cool completely.

Tips

- If you use part-skim ricotta cheese, drain it in a fine-mesh sieve in the sink or set over a bowl for 1 hour so it's not too watery.

- Try using a little lemon extract and some blueberries for a tasty change.

Nutritional Information | Calories: 267 | Total Carbs: 6.2 g | Dietary Fiber: 1.5 g | Protein: 19.2 g | Fat: 18.3 g | Saturated Fat: 11.2 g

Vanilla Blueberry Panna Cotta

Panna cotta is a creamy, smooth Italian custard set with gelatin rather than eggs. I love pairing it with a sweet blueberry sauce. See bottom left of page 192 for photo.

Yield: 2 servings

Prep Time: 4 hours 15 minutes (includes 4 hours to chill)

Cook Time: 15 minutes

Total Time: 4 hours 30 minutes

DAIRY-FREE, EGG-FREE OPTION, NUT-FREE OPTION

FOR PANNA COTTA:

- ¾ cup (175 ml) unsweetened almond or hemp milk (nut-free option)
- ½ cup (120 ml) full-fat coconut milk
- 1¼ teaspoons grass-fed gelatin
- ¾ teaspoon vanilla extract
- Seeds of ½ scraped vanilla bean (optional)
- ⅓ cup (37 g) egg white protein powder
- 2½ tablespoons (20 g) powdered sweetener

FOR BLUEBERRY SAUCE:

- ⅓ cup (50 g) fresh blueberries
- 2 teaspoons water
- 1 tablespoon (8 g) powdered sweetener
- ½ teaspoon grated lemon zest
- ¼ teaspoon glucomannan or xanthan gum

1. Lightly grease two 6-ounce (170 ml) ramekins or bowls.

2. To make the panna cotta: Pour the almond milk and coconut milk into a small saucepan and sprinkle the surface with the gelatin. Let sit for 3 minutes to bloom. Place the pan over medium heat, whisking to dissolve the gelatin. Bring just to a simmer, then remove the pan from the heat. Whisk in the vanilla extract and vanilla bean seeds (if using).

3. In a blender, combine the protein powder and sweetener. Pour in the almond milk mixture. Blend for 10 seconds to combine. Divide the mixture between the 2 ramekins and refrigerate for 4 hours to set.

4. To unmold, set a ramekin in a bowl of hot water (don't let the water come over the top) for 15 to 20 seconds. Place a plate on top and flip over together. Shake the ramekin to loosen. Repeat.

5. To make the blueberry sauce: In a small saucepan over medium-low heat, combine the berries and water. Bring to a simmer and cook until the berries soften and begin to release their juices, about 5 minutes. Remove from the heat and stir in the sweetener and lemon zest. Sprinkle the surface with the glucomannan and whisk vigorously to combine. Spoon the sauce over the panna cotta and serve.

Tips

You can also use Knox gelatin, but you will need only 1 teaspoon. Try raspberries or strawberries in place of the blueberries.

Nutritional Information | Calories: 214 | Total Carbs: 5.7 g | Dietary Fiber: 0.4 g | Protein: 18.7 g | Fat: 13.7 g | Saturated Fat: 11.4 g

Tiramisu Mousse Cups

The classic Italian dessert goes low carb and high protein. Skip the high-carb ladyfingers and just enjoy the creamy tiramisu filling. See bottom right of page 1 for photo.

Yield: 4 servings

Prep Time: 2 hours 20 minutes (includes 2 hours to chill)

Total Time: 2 hours 20 minutes

EGG-FREE, NUT-FREE

1 cup (240 g) high-protein yogurt

⅓ cup (40 g) unflavored protein powder of choice

⅓ cup (43 g) powdered sweetener

4 ounces (115 g) mascarpone cheese, softened

2 teaspoons instant espresso powder

½ teaspoon vanilla extract

1½ tablespoons (25 ml) water

1½ teaspoons grass-fed gelatin

1½ tablespoons (8 g) cocoa powder

½ ounce (14 g) sugar-free dark chocolate

Protein powder options

Just about any protein powder should work here.

1. In a medium-size bowl, whisk the yogurt, protein powder, and sweetener until well combined.

2. In another medium-size bowl, whisk the mascarpone, espresso powder, and vanilla until smooth.

3. In a small microwave-safe bowl, whisk the water and the gelatin. Heat on high power for 30 seconds, then whisk again to dissolve the gelatin. Beat into the yogurt mixture, then fold the yogurt mixture into the mascarpone mixture until no streaks remain.

4. Spoon about one-third of the mousse into 4 small dessert cups. Sprinkle each with a little of the cocoa powder, then spoon another third into the cups and sprinkle with more cocoa powder. Top with the final third of the mixture.

5. Refrigerate for 2 hours to firm up, then use a cheese grater to shave the chocolate over the top of each before serving.

Tips

- If you can't find mascarpone cheese, use cream cheese. You may need to add a little heavy whipping cream to make it thin enough to fold into the yogurt mixture.

- Use a powdered sweetener to avoid grittiness. You can also use concentrated extracts like stevia or monk fruit.

Nutritional Information | Calories: 211 | Total Carbs: 7.3 g | Dietary Fiber: 1.5 g | Protein: 15.7 g | Fat: 15.9 g | Saturated Fat: 8.4 g

Peanut Butter Protein Ice Cream

Ice cream might just be one of my all-time favorite desserts. Being able to enjoy low-carb ice cream that helps me meet my protein goals makes it taste even better!

Yield: 6 servings

Prep Time: 6 hours 20 minutes (includes 6 hours to chill)

Total Time: 6 hours 20 minutes

EGG-FREE, VEGETARIAN

- 1½ cups (338 g) cottage cheese
- ½ cup (60 g) unflavored protein powder
- ½ cup (96 g) allulose granular sweetener
- ⅓ cup (87 g) creamy natural peanut butter
- ½ cup (120 ml) heavy whipping cream
- 3 tablespoons (24 g) powdered sweetener
- ½ teaspoon vanilla extract
- 4 sugar-free peanut butter cups, chopped (optional)

1. In a food processor or high-powered blender, blend the cottage cheese until smooth. Add the protein powder, allulose sweetener, and peanut butter and blend until well combined.

2. In a large bowl, using a handheld electric mixer, beat the cream with the powdered sweetener and vanilla on medium-high speed until it holds stiff peaks. Fold the cottage cheese mixture into the whipped cream until no streaks remain. Stir in the peanut butter cups (if using). Spread the mixture in an airtight container and freeze until firm, 5 to 6 hours.

Tips

- Allulose is useful in low-carb ice cream recipes because it helps keep it from freezing rock solid, but you can use any sweetener as long as it dissolves well. However, you may need to let the ice cream sit on the counter for 5 to 10 minutes before serving to be able to scoop it.

- I used LILY'S Peanut Butter Cups for this ice cream, but you could also simply add some sugar-free chocolate chips.

Protein powder options

Just about any protein powder should work here. I find that plant proteins can have a strong flavor that overpowers the ice cream flavor.

Nutritional Information | Calories: 270 | Total Carbs: 8.6 g | Dietary Fiber: 2.7 g | Protein: 19.3 g | Fat: 19.7 g | Saturated Fat: 10.1 g

Easy Raspberry Frozen Yogurt

Creamy, dreamy, and ready when you are. Whipping up this high-protein frozen yogurt is easy with a little advanced prep work. No ice cream maker necessary!

Yield: 2 servings

Prep Time: 2 hours 10 minutes (includes 2 hours to freeze)

Total Time: 2 hours 10 minutes

EGG-FREE, NUT-FREE, VEGETARIAN

1 cup (240 g) high-protein yogurt, divided

½ cup (70 g) frozen raspberries

¼ cup (30 g) unflavored whey protein powder

3 tablespoons (24 g) powdered sweetener

½ teaspoon vanilla extract

1. Measure out ⅓ cup (80 g) of the yogurt and spoon it into ice cube trays or small silicone molds. Place in the freezer for 2 hours.

2. Once the yogurt is frozen, place the remaining ⅔ cup (160 g) yogurt into a food processor or high-powered blender. Add the frozen raspberries, frozen yogurt cubes, protein powder, sweetener, and vanilla. Blend on high speed until smooth and creamy. You may need to stop to scrape down the sides of the food processor or blender several times to get it to blend smoothly.

3. Serve immediately for a soft-serve consistency or transfer to a freezer-safe container and freeze for another 30 to 60 minutes for a firmer, scoopable consistency.

Tips

- Freezing some of the yogurt in little bite-size pieces first allows the frozen yogurt to have a thicker consistency after blending. It would be more like a smoothie if you tried to blend the yogurt and berries just as they are.

- If the yogurt or protein powder you use is sweetened, you may want to cut back on or omit the added sweetener.

Protein powder options

This recipe should work well with any protein powder. Keep in mind that hemp or other plant-based proteins may change the appearance and flavor.

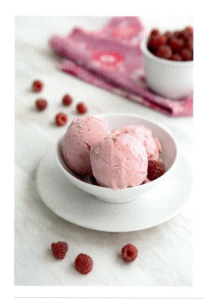

Nutritional Information | Calories: 128 | Total Carbs: 7.1 g | Dietary Fiber: 2 g | Protein: 20.9 g | Fat: 2.2 g | Saturated Fat: 0.5 g

Collagen Fudge Cups

Chocolate fudge that's good for your joints, hair, and skin? Now that's my kind of treat! These are easy to make and store well in the fridge so you can keep them on hand for protein emergencies.

Yield: 9 cups (1 fudge cup per serving)

Prep Time: 2 hours 10 minutes (includes 2 hours to chill)

Total Time: 2 hours 10 minutes

EGG-FREE, NUT-FREE OPTION

⅔ cup (173 g) creamy almond butter

2 ounces (55 g) unsweetened chocolate, chopped

2 tablespoons (28 g) unsalted butter, plus 2 teaspoons, as needed

½ teaspoon vanilla extract

½ cup (56 g) chocolate collagen protein powder

3 tablespoons (24 g) powdered sweetener

Flaked sea salt, for seasoning (optional)

1. Line a standard muffin tin with 9 silicone or parchment paper liners.

2. Set a heatproof bowl over a pan of barely simmering water without allowing the bottom of the bowl to touch the water. In the bowl, combine the almond butter, unsweetened chocolate, and 2 tablespoons (28 g) of the butter, stirring until melted and smooth. Stir in the vanilla. Remove the bowl from the pan.

3. Whisk in the collagen and sweetener until well combined and smooth. If the mixture is overly thick and won't smooth out, add another 1 to 2 teaspoons of butter. Divide the mixture evenly among the prepared muffin cups and sprinkle with sea salt (if using). Refrigerate for 2 hours until firm.

4. Store the cups in an airtight container in the refrigerator for up to 10 days.

Tips

- If you only have plain collagen powder, you may need to add a little cocoa powder (about 1½ teaspoons) and additional sweetener to taste.

- Use any nut or seed butter for this recipe. Try pumpkin seed butter for a nut-free option.

- Use your preferred sweetener here as long as it will dissolve well into the mixture. I recommend a powdered sweetener. I also recommend sifting it before adding it so you don't get any little clumps.

Nutritional Information | Calories: 208 | Total Carbs: 5.3 g | Dietary Fiber: 3 g | Protein: 12.1 g | Fat: 15.3 g | Saturated Fat: 4.9 g

Coconut Candy Bars

If you love Mounds, you'll love these high-protein candy bars. If you don't need these to be nut-free, you can also top them with almonds and turn them into Almond Joy. See top left of page 192 for photo.

Yield: 8 bars (1 bar per serving)

Prep Time: 1 hour 25 minutes (includes 1 hour to freeze)

Total Time: 1 hour 25 minutes

DAIRY-FREE, EGG-FREE OPTION, NUT-FREE

1½ cups (120 g) finely shredded coconut

½ cup (56 g) egg white protein powder

⅓ cup (43 g) powdered sweetener

2 tablespoons (14 g) collagen protein powder

1 tablespoon (7 g) coconut flour

¼ cup (60 ml) full-fat coconut milk

1 teaspoon coconut extract

½ teaspoon vanilla extract

2 ounces (55 g) sugar-free dark chocolate, chopped

½ ounce (14 g) cocoa butter

Protein powder options

Use your favorite protein powder for this recipe. Use whey for an egg-free option.

1. Line a sheet pan with wax paper.

2. In a large bowl, whisk the coconut, egg white protein powder, sweetener, collagen protein powder, and coconut flour to blend.

3. Stir in the coconut milk, coconut extract, and vanilla until well combined. Spoon the mixture into 8 mounds on the prepared pan. Form the mounds into small, flat logs. Freeze for 1 hour.

4. Set a heatproof bowl over a pan of barely simmering water without allowing the bottom of the bowl to touch the water. Place the chopped chocolate and cocoa butter in the bowl and stir until melted and smooth. Remove the bowl from the pan.

5. One at a time, dip the frozen coconut bars into the chocolate, using a fork to toss to coat. Place the coated bars back on the tray to firm up.

6. Store the bars in an airtight container in the refrigerator for up to 10 days.

Tips

- Cocoa butter helps thin the chocolate, allowing you to coat the candy bars more smoothly and evenly. You can use 1½ teaspoons coconut oil instead, but the bars will be more melty at room temperature.

- A little collagen protein gives these bars more chewiness as well as additional protein.

Nutritional Information | Calories: 203 | Total Carbs: 8.1 g | Dietary Fiber: 3.7 g | Protein: 10.4 g | Fat: 16.6 g | Saturated Fat: 13.8 g

Peppermint Patties

There is something so delectable about the combination of peppermint and chocolate. If you love York Peppermint Patties, then these sugar-free protein treats are a must make. See top left of page 1 for photo.

Yield: 12 patties (2 patties per serving)

Prep Time: 2 hours 50 minutes (includes 2 hours 30 minutes to freeze)

Total Time: 2 hours 50 minutes

EGG-FREE, NUT-FREE, VEGETARIAN

4 ounces (115 g) cream cheese, softened

¼ cup (56 g) cottage cheese, blended

½ cup (60 g) unflavored whey protein powder

¼ cup (32 g) powdered sweetener

1 teaspoon peppermint extract

½ teaspoon vanilla extract

3 ounces (85 g) sugar-free dark chocolate, chopped

¾ ounce (21 g) cocoa butter

Protein powder options

You can use egg white protein or plant-based protein for these patties. Just keep in mind that plant proteins may change the color and flavor.

1. Line a sheet pan with wax paper.

2. In a medium bowl, with a handheld mixer, beat the cream cheese and cottage cheese on medium-high speed until creamy, about 1 minute.

3. Add the protein powder, sweetener, peppermint extract, and vanilla and beat until well combined. Using about 1 tablespoon (24 g) per patty, dollop the mixture onto the prepared pan, spreading it into 12 small circles. Alternatively, spoon the mixture into small silicone molds. Freeze for 2 hours until solid.

4. Set a heatproof bowl over a pan of barely simmering water without allowing the bottom of the bowl to touch the water. Place the chopped chocolate and cocoa butter in the bowl and stir until melted and smooth. Remove the bowl from the pan.

5. One at a time, dip the frozen patties into the chocolate, using a fork to toss to coat. Place the patties back on the tray and return to the freezer for 30 minutes to firm up.

6. Store in an airtight container in the refrigerator for up to 5 days.

Tips

- I recommend a bulk powdered sweetener for this recipe, to give it the right consistency without any grittiness.

- Make sure the patties are frozen solid before dipping them in the melted chocolate.

Nutritional Information | Calories: 182 | Total Carbs: 7.4 g | Dietary Fiber: 2.8 g | Protein: 10.7 g | Fat: 13.7 g | Saturated Fat: 8.7 g

Strawberry Lemonade Ice Pops

I make batches of these low-carb ice pops all summer long. They help keep us cool and fueled!

Yield: 5 ice pops (1 ice pop per serving)

Prep Time: 6 hours 10 minutes (includes 6 hours to freeze)

Total Time: 6 hours 10 minutes

DAIRY-FREE, NUT-FREE, VEGETARIAN

- 1 cup (170 g) chopped fresh strawberries
- ¾ cup (175 ml) full-fat coconut milk
- ½ cup (56 g) unflavored egg white protein powder
- ¼ cup (48 g) sweetener, plus more as needed (see Tips)
- 2 teaspoons grated lemon zest
- 2 tablespoons (28 ml) freshly squeezed lemon juice

1. In a blender, combine all of the ingredients and blend until smooth. Taste and adjust the sweetener to your liking. Pour the mixture into 5 ice pop molds, about 3 ounces (85 g) each. Tap the molds lightly on the counter a few times to release any air bubbles.

2. Insert wooden craft sticks about two-thirds of the way into the pops. (The mixture should be thick enough for the sticks to stay in place; if not, freeze the ice pops for 1 hour, then insert the sticks). Freeze for at least 6 hours.

3. To unmold the ice pops, heat some water in a kettle and run it over the outside of the mold you want to release for 5 to 10 seconds. Gently tug the stick to remove the ice pop.

Tips

Use your preferred sweetener here as long as it dissolves well and won't be gritty. I like to use a combination of allulose and erythritol. The allulose keeps the ice pops from freezing rock solid in the freezer.

Protein powder options

This recipe will work well with any protein powder. Keep in mind that plant-based protein may change the color and may have a stronger flavor.

Nutritional Information | Calories: 116 | Total Carbs: 4.7 g | Dietary Fiber: 0.7 g | Protein: 10.1 g | Fat: 7.3 g | Saturated Fat: 6.8 g

CHAPTER 10

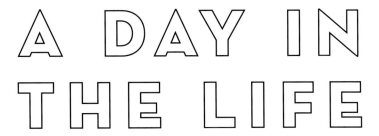

A DAY IN THE LIFE

Increasing your protein and lowering your carbs can seem like a daunting task at times, particularly if you are used to a standard American diet. It can feel like work to meet your protein goals for the day. And you'll sometimes find yourself standing in front of an open fridge or cupboard wondering what you can eat.

Let me reassure that with a little practice, it soon becomes second nature. And as your body adjusts and you gain some energy, lose a little weight, or stabilize your blood sugar (or all of the above!), it becomes ever more enjoyable. If my personal experience is any indication, you may even find you no longer crave the high-carb, low-protein foods you used to love.

To show you what real-life low-carb, high-protein eating looks like, I tracked my food for a few days. Keep in mind that this is not a meal plan, and it is tailored to my individual needs, preferences, and goals.

I am a small-statured woman in her fifties who runs and participates in CrossFit-style workouts. I crave variety, and I also like to utilize leftovers for easy breakfasts and lunches. I don't have a huge appetite in one sitting, so I prefer to break things into smaller meals with snacks. I routinely make a morning cappuccino with almond milk, cream, and collagen. And I love dessert!

Day 1

6 a.m. pre-workout snack	Protein muffin: 181 calories, 11 g protein, 6 g carbs
9 a.m. post-workout breakfast	Leftover Korean Beef and Broccoli (page 166): 408 calories, 30 g protein, 7 g carbs
9:30 a.m. collagen cappuccino	130 calories, 10 g protein, 0.5 g carbs
12:30 p.m. lunch	Green salad with cucumber, avocado, canned tuna, sesame oil dressing: 339 calories, 26 g protein, 7 g carbs
3 p.m. afternoon snack	⅓ cup (34 g) salted pecans: 228 calories, 3 g protein, 5 g carbs
6 p.m. dinner	Chicken Chile Verde (page 129): 311 calories, 35 g protein, 7 g carbs
6:45 p.m. dessert	Deep-Dish Brownie (page 197): 201 calories, 16 g protein, 7 g carbs
Exercise	CrossFit class with weight lifting and physical conditioning as well as a 4-mile (6.4 km) walk
Daily totals	1798 calories, 131 g protein, 39.5 g carbs

Day 2

6 a.m. pre-workout snack	Carrot Cake Protein Bites (page 114): 211 calories, 9 g protein, 6 g carbs
9 a.m. post-workout breakfast	Turkey Breakfast Sausage (page 48), 1 fried egg, ⅓ cup (42 g) raspberries: 360 calories, 28 g protein, 7 g carbs
9:30 a.m. collagen cappuccino	130 calories, 10 g protein, 0.5 g carbs
12:30 p.m. lunch	Garlic Parmesan Chicken Skewers (page 152) with cucumber and red bell pepper: 337 calories, 28 g protein, 7 g carbs
3:30 p.m. afternoon snack	⅓ cup (75 g) cottage cheese: 53 calories, 9 g protein, 2 g carbs
6:30 p.m. dinner	Easy Steak Fajitas (page 165) with cauliflower rice: 330 calories, 26 g protein, 10 g carbs
7 p.m. dessert	1 scoop homemade keto ice cream: 285 calories, 1.5 g protein, 2.3 g carbs
Exercise	2-mile (3.2 km) walk with the dog, 4-mile (6.4 km) run
Daily totals	1706 calories, 111.5 g protein, 35 g carbs

Day 3

Pre-workout snack	None
8:30 a.m. post-workout breakfast	1 Denver Omelet Cup (page 47), 1 Italian chicken sausage (Whole Foods brand), leftover sautéed veggies: 352 calories, 25 g protein, 7 g carbs
9:30 a.m. collagen cappuccino	130 calories, 10 g protein, 0.5 g carbs
12 p.m. lunch	Salad with cucumber, avocado, grilled chicken, walnut oil dressing: 375 calories, 32 g protein, 7 g carbs
3 p.m. afternoon snack	Cold-brew coffee with heavy cream, ½-ounce (14 g) square low-carb chocolate: 140 calories, 2 g protein, 5 g carbs
6 p.m. dinner	Teriyaki Salmon (page 183) with roasted broccoli: 359 calories, 30 g protein, 7 g carbs
6:30 p.m. dessert	Homemade low-carb cheesecake bar: 260 calories, 5 g protein, 6 g carbs
Exercise	CrossFit class with weight lifting and physical conditioning, 3-mile (4.8 km) walk
Daily totals	1616 calories, 104 g protein, 32.5 g carbs

Quick Protein Boosts

Sometimes even the most carefully laid plans go awry. No matter how much planning you do, you will have days when you struggle to meet your protein targets. Maybe you had a long day at work and don't have the time or energy to cook. Maybe you had a meal out with friends where the protein options were scarce. Maybe you open the fridge to discover that someone ate the yummy protein you cooked for yourself (I might be speaking from experience here).

First step, don't panic. It happens to all of us at least once in a while. Not hitting your protein target for one day won't derail your progress or throw you into severe catabolism.

There are plenty of delicious ways to get a quick hit of protein when you need one. They can be stand-alone snacks or added to a full meal to boost the overall protein content. I like to use protein desserts or snacks to round out a lighter meal and provide a full complement of amino acids.

Cottage cheese: Once the domain of 1980s-era fad diets, this funny curdy stuff is making a comeback. It packs a serious protein punch (½ cup, or 113 g, has up to 14 grams), and is a tasty addition to granola, eggs, and salads. I've discovered that I even like it plain!

Dessert: Have I mentioned I have a sweet tooth? I eat a little bit of dessert every day. So I consider it a nutritional bonus if my dessert contains a little protein too. Since I eat it soon after I finish my dinner, I often count it as part of my dinner protein totals.

Hard-boiled eggs: These days, you can easily find hard-boiled eggs ready to go at the grocery store. I like to eat them on their own, with a little salt and pepper. They are also great chopped up on salad or sliced and arranged on a piece of protein toast.

Meat sticks: Individual pepperoni and jerky sticks are a great protein snack, especially when you're on the go. Read the labels because some brands and varieties have added sugar. I like the uncured meat sticks from brands like Chomps or Paleovalley.

Peanut butter: A scoop of peanut butter on a spoon may be the ultimate childhood snack, but it's a great way to add a touch of protein into your diet. Most natural peanut butters have 7 or 8 grams of protein per 2-tablespoon (32 g) serving, and almond butter is about the same.

Protein balls: I love keeping homemade protein balls, like the Snickerdoodle Protein Bites (page 113), in my fridge for quick snacks. They are easy to make and can last up to 10 days in a covered container. When my main meal is a little light on protein, I use things like this to meet the 25-gram protein threshold.

Protein-enhanced yogurt: Greek yogurt is relatively high in protein, but there are now many brands with additional protein. Read the labels because some may have added sugar. I tend to stick with the plain varieties, as they often have fewer carbs.

Pumpkin seeds and hemp seeds: These high-protein, low-carb seeds are a great way to add a bit of protein to a meal. Sprinkle them on salads or add them to yogurt for added crunch. Shelled, roasted pumpkin seeds also come in some great flavors you can enjoy straight from the bag.

Tuna pouches: Many brands of canned tuna now offer single-serve pouches that have about 20 grams of protein. They can be plain or flavored, so check the nutritional label to make sure it doesn't contain added carbohydrates.

REFERENCES

Agergaard, Jakob, et al. "Even or skewed dietary protein distribution is reflected in the whole-body protein net-balance in healthy older adults: A randomized controlled trial." *Clinical Nutrition* 42, no. 6 (June 2023): 899. doi:10.1016/j.clnu.2023.04.004

Aragon, Alan A., and Brad J. Schoenfeld. "Nutrient timing revisited: is there a post-exercise anabolic window?" *Journal of the International Society of Sports Nutrition* 10, no. 5 (January 2013): 5. doi:10.1186/1550-2783-10-5

Beaudry, Kayleigh M., and Michaela C. Devries. "Nutritional Strategies to Combat Type 2 Diabetes in Aging Adults: The Importance of Protein." *Frontiers in Nutrition* 6 (August 2019): 138. doi:10.3389/fnut.2019.00138

Bopp, Melanie J., et al. "Lean Mass Loss Is Associated with Low Protein Intake during Dietary-Induced Weight Loss in Postmenopausal Women." *Journal of the Academy of Nutrition and Dietetics* 108, no. 7 (July 2008): 1216. doi:10.1016/j.jada.2008.04.017

Carbone, John W., and Stefan M. Pasiakos. "Dietary Protein and Muscle Mass: Translating Science to Application and Health Benefit." *Nutrients* 11, no. 5 (May 2019): 1136. doi:10.3390/nu11051136

Coelho-Junior, Hélio José, et al. "Protein Intake and Sarcopenia in Older Adults: A Systematic Review and Meta-Analysis." *International Journal of Environmental Research and Public Health* 19, no. 14 (July 2022): 8718. doi:10.3390/ijerph19148718

Chow, Lisa S., et al. "Mechanism of insulin's anabolic effect on muscle: measurements of muscle protein synthesis and breakdown using aminoacyl-tRNA and other surrogate measures." *American Journal of Physiology* 291, no. 4 (October 2006): E729. doi:10.1152/ajpendo.00003.2006

Gannon, Mary C., et al. "An increase in dietary protein improves the blood glucose response in persons with type 2 diabetes." *The American Journal of Clinical Nutrition* 78, no. 4 (October 2003): 734. doi:10.1093/ajcn/78.4.734

Gannon, Mary C., et al. "Effect of Protein Ingestion on the Glucose Appearance Rate in People with Type 2 Diabetes." *The Journal of Clinical Endocrinology & Metabolism* 86, no. 3 (March 2001): 1040. doi:10.1210/jcem.86.3.7263

Gregorio, L., et al. "Adequate dietary protein is associated with better physical performance among post-menopausal women 60–90 years." *The Journal of Nutrition, Health, and Aging* 18, no. 2 (February 2014): 155. doi:10.1007/s12603-013-0391-2

Hruby, Adela, et al. "Protein Intake and Functional Integrity in Aging: The Framingham Heart Study Offspring." *The Journals of Gerontology: Series A* 75, no 1 (January 2020): 123. doi:10.1093/gerona/gly201

Hudson, Joshua L., et al. "Protein Distribution and Muscle-Related Outcomes: Does the Evidence Support the Concept?" *Nutrients* 12, no. 5 (May 2020): 1441. doi:10.3390/nu12051441

Isanejad, Masoud, et al. "Dietary protein intake is associated with better physical function and muscle strength among elderly women." *British Journal of Nutrition* 115, no. 7 (April 2016): 1281. doi:10.1017/S000711451600012X

Kim, Il-Young, et al. "Quantity of dietary protein intake, but not pattern of intake, affects net protein balance primarily through differences in protein synthesis in older adults." *American Journal of Physiology* 308, no. 1 (January 2015): E21. doi:10.1152/ajpendo.00382.2014

Kerstetter, Jane E., Anne M. Kenny, and Karl L. Insogna. "Dietary protein and skeletal health: a review of recent human research." *Current Opinion in Lipidology* 22, no. 1 (February 2011): 16. doi:10.1097/MOL.0b013e3283419441

Leidy, Heather J., et al. "The role of protein in weight loss and maintenance." *The American Journal of Clinical Nutrition* 101, no. 6 (June 2015): 1320S. doi:10.3945/ajcn.114.084038

Lesgards, Jean-François. "Benefits of Whey Proteins on Type 2 Diabetes Mellitus Parameters and Prevention of Cardiovascular Diseases." *Nutrients* 15, no. 5 (March 2023): 1294. doi:10.3390/nu15051294

Moon, Jaecheol, and Gwanpyo Koh. "Clinical Evidence and Mechanisms of High-Protein Diet-Induced Weight Loss." *Journal of Obesity & Metabolic Syndrome* 29, no. 3 (September 2020): 166. doi:10.7570/jomes20028

Moore, Daniel R., et al. "Protein ingestion to stimulate myofibrillar protein synthesis requires greater relative protein intakes in healthy older versus younger men." *The Journals of Gerontology: Series A* 70, no. 1 (January 2015): 57. doi:10.1093/gerona/glu103

Morton, Robert W., et al. "A systematic review, meta-analysis and meta-regression of the effect of protein supplementation on resistance training-induced gains in muscle mass and strength in healthy adults." *British Journal of Sports Medicine* 52, no. 6 (March 2018): 376. doi:10.1136/bjsports-2017-097608

Paddon-Jones, Douglas, et al. "Protein, weight management, and satiety." *The American Journal of Clinical Nutrition* 87, no. 5 (May 2008): 1558S. doi:10.1093/ajcn/87.5.1558S

Paddon-Jones, Douglas, et al. "Protein and healthy aging." *The American Journal of Clinical Nutrition* 101, no. 6 (June 2015): 1339S. doi:10.3945/ajcn.114.084061

Park, Young-Min, et al. "A High-Protein Breakfast Induces Greater Insulin and Glucose-Dependent Insulinotropic Peptide Responses to a Subsequent Lunch Meal in Individuals with Type 2 Diabetes." *The Journal of Nutrition* 145, no. 3 (March 2015): 452. doi:10.3945/jn.114.202549

Park, Sanghee, et al. "Metabolic Evaluation of the Dietary Guidelines' Ounce Equivalents of Protein Food Sources in Young Adults: A Randomized Controlled Trial." *The Journal of Nutrition* 151, no. 5 (May 2021): 1190. doi:10.1093/jn/nxaa401

Pasiakos, Stefan M., Harris R. Lieberman, and Victor L. Fulgoni 3rd. "Higher-Protein Diets Are Associated with Higher HDL Cholesterol and Lower BMI and Waist Circumference in US Adults." *The Journal of Nutrition* 145, no. 3 (March 2015): 605. doi:10.3945/jn.114.205203

Paul, Cristiana, Suzane Leser, and Steffen Oesser. "Significant Amounts of Functional Collagen Peptides Can Be Incorporated in the Diet While Maintaining Indispensable Amino Acid Balance." *Nutrients* 11, no. 5 (May 2019): 1079. doi:10.3390/nu11051079

Pesta, Dominik H., and Varman T. Samuel. "A high-protein diet for reducing body fat: mechanisms and possible caveats." *Nutrition & Metabolism*, 11 (November 2014): 53. doi:10.1186/1743-7075-11-53

Phillips, Stuart M., Stephanie Chevalier, and Heather J. Leidy. "Protein 'requirements' beyond the RDA: implications for optimizing health." *Applied Physiology, Nutrition, and Metabolism* 41, no. 5 (May 2016): 565. doi:10.1139/apnm-2015-0550

Pinckaers, Philippe J. M., et al. "The Anabolic Response to Plant-Based Protein Ingestion." *Sports Medicine* 51, Suppl 1 (September 2021): 59. doi:10.1007/s40279-021-01540-8

Trommelen, Jorn, et al. "The anabolic response to protein ingestion during recovery from exercise has no upper limit in magnitude and duration in vivo in humans." *Cell Reports Medicine* 4, no. 12 (December 2023): 322. doi:10.1016/j.xcrm.2023.101324

Tricò, Domenico, et al. "Effects of Low-Carbohydrate versus Mediterranean Diets on Weight Loss, Glucose Metabolism, Insulin Kinetics and β-Cell Function in Morbidly Obese Individuals." *Nutrients* 13, no. 4 (April 2021): 1345. doi:10.3390/nu13041345

Vasdev, Sudesh, and Jennifer Stuckless. "Antihypertensive effects of dietary protein and its mechanisms." *International Journal of Angiology* 19, no. 1 (Spring 2010): e7. doi:10.1055/s-0031-1278362

Volek, Jeff S., et al. "Expert consensus on nutrition and lower-carbohydrate diets: An evidence- and equity-based approach to dietary guidance." *Frontiers in Nutrition* 11 (February 2024): 1376098. doi:10.3389/fnut.2024.1376098

Yongsoon, Park, Choi Jeong-Eun, and Hwang Hwan-Sik. "Protein supplementation improves muscle mass and physical performance in undernourished prefrail and frail elderly subjects: a randomized, double-blind, placebo-controlled trial." *The American Journal of Clinical Nutrition* 108, no. 5 (November 2018): 1026. doi:10.1093/ajcn/nqy214

ACKNOWLEDGMENTS

Bringing a cookbook to life is no small feat and requires the time, effort, expertise, and support of so many individuals. Where do I even start?

Thank you to Jill Alexander of Quarto for reaching out and offering me this project. It dovetailed so perfectly with my own journey, I could hardly say no. And to the rest of the team at Fair Winds Press, especially Mary Cassells and Kelly Desabrais, thank you for sanding down the rough edges of my work and giving it polish.

To my wonderful husband, Tim, who has been on this cookbook journey with me seven times and still loves me, thank you for your infinite patience and your willingness to eat all of my experiments (successful or not!).

To Laura Bashar, for your recipe testing and proofreading expertise, and to Stephanie Kenyon, for holding down the fort on social media and always cheering me on. You are both so very much appreciated!

To all my wonderful and supportive friends who play the role of taste-testers, thank you for letting me bombard your tastebuds. A special shout-out to the crew at Intrepid Athletics for always being so enthused whenever I bring in samples and treats.

Finally, to the amazing readers and fans of All Day I Dream About Food—some of whom have been on this journey with me for over a decade—I could not do this without you. You are the reason I keep going, even when the obstacles seem insurmountable. I feel ever so lucky to have discovered this world where food can be both wholesome sustenance and celebration.

ABOUT THE AUTHOR

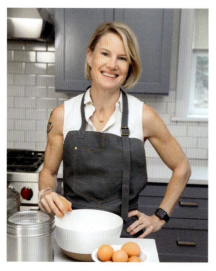

CAROLYN KETCHUM is the self-proclaimed mad genius behind the popular low-carb website All Day I Dream About Food, and the bestselling author of multiple cookbooks, including *The Ultimate Guide to Keto Baking*. Her devoted following includes dieters, diabetics, fitness enthusiasts, and those simply trying to embrace a healthier lifestyle. Her work has been featured in *Women's Health*, Glamour.com, *Good Housekeeping*, and *Muscle & Fitness Hers*, among others.

Carolyn's mission is to prove that special diets need not be boring or restrictive and that healthy eating is about more than just sustenance. She wants to show the world that low-carb, high-protein dishes can be just as good as *or better* than their sugar- and flour-filled counterparts. The absence of guilt is the special sauce that makes her recipes extra delicious.

Carolyn has a master's degree in anthropology and early human evolution and an extensive background in higher education administration. She lives in Portland, Oregon, with her husband, three children, and Taco, the fluffy Australian Shepherd.

INDEX